The ABC's of Health

Your Path To Greatness

By Dr. Aaron D. Tressler B.S., D.C.

ISBN –9781494737658

Printed in the United States of America

Disclaimer: All of the information contained in ABC's of Health is provided with the understanding that readers accept responsibility for their health and well-being. This publication makes no attempt to diagnose or treat conditions or diseases, nor is it meant to be a substitute for the advice of a competent health care professional.

Tressler Chiropractic
4241 William Penn Highway
Murrysville, Pa 15668
724-327-5665
www.DrADT.com
www.DrADTweightloss.com

Call For Your Complimentary Consultation

CONTENTS

ABC's of Health

When I first met Dr. Aaron Tressler eight years ago we were in Dallas, Texas at a chiropractic seminar since then, he has been not only a friend, but also a chiropractic brother. We are constantly pushing each other to serve more and help more people. In his first chapter he speaks of attitude and the power of positivity. Dr. Tressler is one of the most positive people I know, always looking at the glass half full, instead of half empty. I believe if we all lived that way we be in a happier place and have less need for the many medications people are prescribed for various 'labels' they are given.

Dr. Tressler has an undying passion for helping people truly get healthy and saving people's lives in the process. Dr. Tressler 'walks the walk of health,' what I mean is, he just doesn't speak it and preach it, he lives it. There are too many doctors out there living in a contradiction to health, telling you to do something, however they aren't doing it.

I remember sharing a hotel room with Dr. Tressler at conference in Philadelphia and he pulls out a snack bag. When I think of a snack bag, I am thinking maybe some chips, granola bars or something like that. He pulls out cherry tomatoes and almonds. He also made me get up early and run with him even though I hate running. This is just one of many ways he lives the lifestyle that he speaks about in this book.

He often speaks of his father dying at a young age of a heart attack and that his father never saw him graduate from college. Dr. Tressler strongly feels that if his father had been given the information presented in this book, he would still be here today. Dr. Tressler's passion and love for his father is a huge driving force to make sure there aren't other kids losing their fathers or mothers before their God-given years.

This book captures the spirit of Dr. Tressler in both a simple message of how to live, but also captures the spiritual side of health. I often speak of B.J. Palmer's quote in my practice, "The power that made the body, heals the body." This book will allow you to truly embrace this quote and respect your body and understand that when God designed us, we were designed for greatness, not sickness or disease. Our body is designed to run itself and fight any and all disease if it is functioning properly. Dr. Tressler's last chapter talks about what controls all functions of the body and exactly how your body works. I am a firm believer that with knowledge comes power. Learning the ABC's to health will elevate your consciousness of health and allow you to make a massive shift towards getting healthy and staying healthy. However, just reading this book alone will not make the shift, you MUST TAKE ACTION.

I am honored to have this opportunity to introduce a chiropractic brother, a mentor, and a good friend, but more importantly a chiropractor that truly cares about his "flock" or his people. Dr. Tressler lives the lifestyle that he speaks of in this book.

TAKE ACTION, Dr. John Brouse, D.C.

Brouse Family Chiropractic, Ebensburg, PA

Thank God I found Dr. Tressler or he found me.....

I knew fairly early that I wanted to be a chiropractor. Growing up I was never a fan of medication; it simply did not make sense to me. Fortunately, my family wasn't quick to turn to medicine. I began receiving chiropractic adjustments at a very early age when my mother began getting treatment. When she was examined, Dr. Rich could tell that she had been involved in a car accident years earlier and accurately predicted the sinus troubles she experienced even though it was not the reason for her seeking care at the time. Through chiropractic care, her sinus troubles were resolved, as were both of my brothers' ear infections.

I first noticed chiropractic's impact on my health in high school while participating in sports. At times I would find it difficult to catch my breath after running sprints. It intrigued me to discover these episodes resolved after getting adjusted. This is when I decided I wanted to be a chiropractor. I now know what I was experiencing was exercise induced asthma, and if my family was the type to seek medical treatment first, I would have been given an inhaler to depend on, rather than removing the nerve interference that was causing my lungs to not function optimally!

Early in my chiropractic career I learned that not all chiropractors are the same. Some choose to focus solely on body mechanics and pain relief. Some of these chiropractors were even responsible for my education, teaching future chiropractors that cancer patients should not be adjusted. This never made sense to me since I had my own experience with optimizing the body's healing potential with chiropractic, if anyone needed adjusted; it was someone whose immune system was so damaged that they suffered with cancer!

After graduating, the first 2 practices I joined talked about optimizing the nervous system, but didn't quite practice that way. They put a major emphasis on abiding by insurance coverage and making recommendations based upon that coverage. As insurance coverage approaches health in a mechanistic way, rather than a vitalistic way, it wasn't often that I saw patients realize the true benefits of chiropractic.

Those practice experiences brought me to Dr. Tressler, I was looking for the chiropractic I knew as a child, seeing health restored, rather than using chiropractic as a fix for headaches, neck pain and back pain. As a former headache sufferer, I do recognize the impact chronic pain has on one's life, but I knew chiropractic could offer that and MORE when utilized appropriately.

When first seeing his practice I knew it was something different due to the large number of children and families who were adjusted. Not all of these people were sick, nor were they when they began care. But Dr. Tressler was able to teach them the value of optimizing their nervous system regularly to maximize life, rather than utilizing chiropractic as a treatment for an ache approved by their insurance company.

During my time in his office, I've witnessed many of the miracles of chiropractic: improved hearing and seeing; asthma, allergies gone; kids no longer suffering each winter with colds and ear infections; infants no longer "needing" acid reflux medication; Multiple Sclerosis lesions "diminishing to resolve"; *cancer* disappearing without chemo or radiation, but by simply implementing a healthy lifestyle; and countless people NEVER experiencing any of these things because they've decided to get their spine checked and keep it healthy before a crisis hits. All the things I always intuitively knew were possible, I'm finally able to witness on a daily basis, and take part in helping people achieve!

This book will lead you down a path of greatness if you allow it. But you must ACT and follow the ABC's to health.

Stephanie Barto DC

Associate Chiropractor
Tressler Chiropractic
4241 William Penn Highway
Murrysville, PA 15668
Phone: (724) 327-5665
www.DrADT.com
www.Facebook.com/TresslerChiropractic

ABC's of Health

A = Attitude
B = Behavior
C = Chiropractic

Introduction

Today's search for health and vitality is far-reaching. We see ads and reports on every television station, radio shows, e-mails, Facebook posts, and even drug companies are reporting that they have the answer to all your health concerns. Overwhelming to say the least.

So, where do you start? Whom do you believe? Who's right and who's wrong? What will happen to your health in the next year, five years, and into your senior years if you follow their advice? This book is intended to give you a **foundation** for your health because without a proper foundation, your house will crumble under the stress.

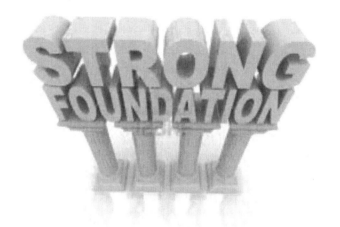

Therefore everyone who hears these words of Mine and puts them into practice is like a wise man who built his house on the rock. The rain came down, the streams rose, and the winds blew and beat against that house; yet it did not fall, because it had its foundation on the rock. But everyone who hears these words of Mine and does not put them into practice is like a foolish man who built his house on sand. The rain came down, the streams rose, and the winds blew and beat against the house, and it fell with a great crash (Matthew 7:24-27).

Jesus' words here are very powerful. The right words are always powerful, and I do suggest that if you follow the right words I'll speak to you through this book and put them into practice, you will build a strong foundation for your health. It takes simple but powerful principles of health to make a difference. Health will not come from the next discovery of a specific plant that will remove all the fat away from your body. You won't find true health in the next new herb or drug but in sound foundational principles – back to the basics. Powerful health comes from doing simple steps, ABC, over and over. Simple may not seem strong enough and doesn't have the pretty packaging or WOW factor that go along with marketing ads, but this simple book about the ACB's to health will transform your health and your life.

If the foundations be destroyed, what can the righteous do? (Psalm 11:3)

I'll begin by asking you a few simple questions: If you were to walk into your kitchen for breakfast tomorrow morning and notice that one of your kitchen chairs only had one leg, would you sit on that chair? I would hope not. If that chair had only two legs, would you sit on it? Still too risky? How about three legs? I don't think so. Disaster is still impending. It's still a broken chair!

If you answered those questions the way I did, I'd say that you have common sense and no desire to hurt yourself; so, as I speak to you throughout this book, I'm going to assume those two things: that you have common sense and that you do not want to harm yourself.

Proceeding from those two assumptions, I'm going to talk about your health by appealing to your common sense and the fact that you value your life. I'm also going to address your health from basic foundational principles that, when neglected, will put your health and life in jeopardy, like balancing on a three-legged chair.

Before we go there, however, please put your attention back on the Biblical verse noted above: *If the foundations be destroyed, what can the righteous do?* Preachers have applied this verse to our spiritual foundation which we need to keep sure and strong in our lives through spiritual disciplines such as reading God's word, prayer, church attendance, and giving, but there's also a principle here that applies in the natural. You see, if there's any instability in any area of your life, failure is imminent unless you work on those parts of the foundation that are unstable – one or perhaps all of the supportive "legs."

Okay, let's look at your health as a chair having four legs: right thinking, good nutrition, consistent exercise, and chiropractic. Do you feel safe sitting on that chair? Based on my forty-seven years on this earth and my nineteen years of professional experience, I promise you that these are the four legs that you absolutely must pay attention to in order to shore up the foundation of true health. If that foundation is destroyed, there's not much you can do, and, sad to say, your destiny is premature death, probably preceded by some daily existence in a nursing home.

But there's good news! We've already determined that you're not the kind of person who sits on broken chairs. You have common sense, and you don't want to hurt yourself; so, I know I can teach you and you can learn. Now, let's move on, shore up the foundation, and see how you can repair and maintain any of those broken or wobbly legs.

For it is written: I will destroy the wisdom of the wise; the intelligence of the intelligent I will frustrate (1 Corinthians 1:19). But God chose the foolish things of the world to shame the wise; God chose the weak things of the world to shame the strong (1 Corinthians 1:27).

The above verses speak of things that the world perceives as foolish and weak because they are simple. The principles you'll learn in this book are, in reality, neither foolish nor weak but so simple that many people overlook them. Folks are constantly looking for the magic pill, the BIG discovery in the lab, or the one exercise that will make it all happen – the shiny package! The ABC's of health are not what the pharmaceutical companies are promoting.

Their ABC's go something like this:

A = Antacids
B = By-pass surgery
C = Cholesterol drugs

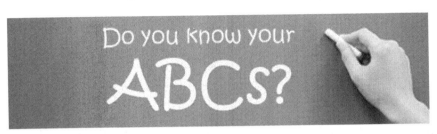

I won't go through their entire alphabet, but I'm sure you get my point. Sad to say, most Americans believe in and live by the pharmaceutical alphabet without even questioning where this is taking them. I was one of those guys, too. In my teen years, as allergies kicked in, I got allergy shots and took over-the-counter medication like candy. As my sinuses were congested, I took nasal spray daily and several times a day when needed. As my stomach pain increased, along with chronic stress-related diarrhea, I lived off Pepto-Bismol. I was heading down the wrong path, and those medications never really did help, but that's all I knew.

I haven't met a single person who wants to live on medication. Most think that they HAVE TO live on it, that there is no other way, or that a natural approach is too expensive, too much work, or ineffective. Our society of "feel good" people prefers easy-to-pop pills that ultimately lead to destruction.

There is a way that seems right to a man, but in the end it leads to death (Proverbs 14:12).

That's a dismal thought, but I remember that you have common sense, that you don't want to harm yourself, and that you value your life; so, let's discover the principles that were designed by God to maintain your health from birth to a good old age. God designed these principles to return your body to health if it has been malfunctioning and to keep it healthy. They work whether you are tall or short, male or female, young or old. They work because they are truth.

Dear friend, I pray that you may enjoy good health and that all may go well with you, even as your soul is getting along well (3 John 1:2).

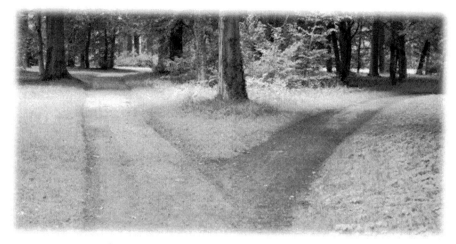

A New Path = A New You!

Chapter 1

ATTITUDE

It all starts here. Without a proper attitude, an attitude of learning, an attitude of gratefulness, an attitude of common sense, all else will fall short. Having a positive attitude can make all the difference. Having an attitude of Christ-like behavior is the most powerful.

You were taught, with regard to your former way of life, to put off your old self, which is being corrupted by its deceitful desires; to be made new in the attitude of your minds; and to put on the new self, created to be like God in true righteousness and holiness (Ephesians 4:22-24).

Our former way of life could be identified as the way the world thinks and behaves. We are taught from birth that shots are necessary for both defending against disease and being allowed to attend school. Doctors taught us to take a pill for every ill. This isn't a principle. It's an attitude, a learned attitude and behavior that must change, and the change begins with a new mind-set that you can be healthy without drugs and surgery at every turn of a health crisis. It begins with believing that your Father created you for health, not sickness.

So God created man in His own image, in the image of God He created him; male and female He created them (Genesis 1:27).

You were not created in the image of your parents, aunts, uncles, or even great grandparents. You were created in the image of God. This should give you hope. If you and I were created in God's image, how would this look? How would you look and feel? Would you need drugs to get over a cold? Would you be obese and unable to climb a flight of stairs without your heart pounding through your chest? Would your knees wear out and need to be replaced? Would you end up in a nursing home, wearing a diaper and having no strength to feed yourself?

Created in the image of God, how should you look and feel? Does your current health status add up to that image, or do you have some work to do? Yes, I did say work. You will work at being healthy or work at being sick. Both take time and money – your choice how that time and money are spent.

Commit to the Lord whatever you do, and your plans will succeed (Proverbs 16:3).

Lazy hands make a man poor, but diligent hands bring wealth (Proverbs 10:4).

He who works his land will have abundant food, but he who chases fantasies lacks judgment (Proverbs 12:11).

Work yields results, and the work begins with commitment to a right attitude:

1. Commit to an attitude that you will win.
2. Commit to an attitude that you don't need medication and surgery to succeed.
3. Commit to an attitude that, made in God's image, you are made with power to heal.
4. Commit to an attitude of strength, not fear.

Drugs and drug companies continue to scare people to death. That is what leads to so many medications.

For God did not give us a spirit of timidity (fearful and hesitant), but a spirit of power, of love and of self-discipline (2 Timothy 1:7).

Get that verse in your memory bank. Commit it to memory, and use it for your daily battles. When we live in fear, we live in weakness. You have powerful, God-given strength to heal and to overcome. Believe in that and hold on to its truth.

Psalm 23: *Even though I walk through the valley of the shadow of death, I will fear no evil, for You are with me (Verse 4).* Many of us are going through a valley right now, will be heading into a valley, or just came out of a valley. As you go through these life challenges, stay strong and do not fear. This does not mean, do nothing. You must work at your health and work at success in life. You must believe that what I'm telling you about attitude is true. Your belief will activate you to do the correct behavior day in and day out and win each battle. Be a winner – not a loser! Your beliefs have all to do with your outcome.

Your mind and what you believe will have a strong impact on your results.

WARNING: CHALLENGES AHEAD – STAY STRONG!

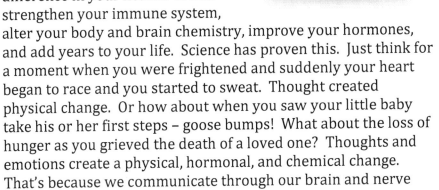

Positive Attitude

Your positive attitude will make a difference in your health. It will strengthen your immune system, alter your body and brain chemistry, improve your hormones, and add years to your life. Science has proven this. Just think for a moment when you were frightened and suddenly your heart began to race and you started to sweat. Thought created physical change. Or how about when you saw your little baby take his or her first steps – goose bumps! What about the loss of hunger as you grieved the death of a loved one? Thoughts and emotions create a physical, hormonal, and chemical change. That's because we communicate through our brain and nerve system, systems that are far superior to all others. I'll tell you more about that later, but for now, consider the research:

1. "At Harvard University, women in mind-body support groups for infertility conceive 44% of the time (as opposed to expected 8 – 10% rate [Domar et al., 2000] and 80% of men with hypertension in mind-body groups are able to decrease their

medication, while 16% are able to stop their antihypertensive medication entirely (Friedman et al., 1992)."

2. "Other studies in the diseases of arthritis (Lorig, 1993), acquired immune deficiency syndrome (AIDS) (Cole et al., 1997), chronic pain (Caudill et al., 1991), as well as for the condition of insomnia (Jacobs et al, 1996), have revealed the benefits of mind-body group skills programs on the health of individuals involved."

3. "At the University of Rochester, Robert Ader, Ph.D., Hon.Doc. Sc., showed that it was possible to classically condition the immune systems of mice."

4. "Meyer Friedman, M.D., studied more than 1000 postmyocardial infarct patients and showed that introducing behavioral counseling altered type-A behavior and reduced cardiac morbidity significantly (Friedman et al., 1984)."

5. "Studies of Harold Koenig, M.D., M.H.Sc., and the late David Larson, M.D., M.S.P.H., at Duke University have proved how spiritual belief increases longevity and protects against illness (Helm et al., 2000; Larson et al., 2000)."

If you Google how your mind affects your health, you will come up with over 24,700,000 results! There is a connection; therefore, as we move towards practical steps that you will apply, and you see how powerfully your body will respond, you must be strong in your beliefs and must want this change for best results. You see, there is nothing more destructive than a negative attitude. Your attitude puts you in motion.

Finally, brothers and sisters, whatever is true, whatever is noble, whatever is right, whatever is pure, whatever is lovely, whatever is admirable – if anything is excellent or praiseworthy – think about such things (Philippians 4:8).

That would be a good start! It's not easy to do, but you must remind yourself daily of positive things, and especially throughout the day, when your mind gets weak, you think negative thoughts, and things start to crumble. You need to stay strong, and it begins with how you think.

Optimist vs. Pessimist

Your psychology can be just as important to your health and well-being as exercise and eating right. There is an entire science on positive thinking: "If you can dream it, then you can achieve it. You will get all you want in life if you help enough other people get what they want" (Zig Ziglar).

If you have ever read anything written by Zig, you will remember this quote. Zig inspired me to dream big. His books, well worth reading, teach that optimism believes big and embraces challenges with a confidence in their positive outcome. Challenges do occur, but how you react to them and the knowledge you gain through them makes all the difference.

Tough? Yes! But you have the strength to endure. *No temptation has overtaken you except what is common to mankind. And God is faithful; He will not let you be tempted beyond what you can bear. But when you are tempted, He will also provide a way out so that you can endure it*
(1 Corinthians 10:13).

That famous verse simply means that God doesn't give us more than we can handle. I have heard, thousands of times, people responding like this: "But it sure feels like He's trying!" Those folks just don't realize that we are capable of surviving through a crisis and becoming stronger. They lack optimism, the knowing that we will all go through some tough challenges and that we will endure. Through those challenges, we either become stronger or broken, depending on our attitude.

Do not grieve, for the joy of the Lord is your strength (Nehemiah 8:10).

Be strong, and let your heart take courage, all you who wait for the Lord (Psalm 31:24).

God is our refuge and strength, an ever-present help in trouble (Psalm 46:1).

So stay strong through your challenges. Believe in great things to come, and never, ever give up hope. It's up to you to re-wire your mind. Consider this: Only twenty-five percent of a person's optimism may be hardwired in his genes, according to some studies. Science suggests that the greater part of an optimistic outlook can be acquired with right instruction. A study of college freshmen, done by Seligman, had pessimistic students take a twelve-week optimism training course which included exercises like writing a letter of gratitude and reading it aloud to someone. Following the course, these freshmen were less likely to visit the student health center for illnesses during the next four years than pessimistic peers who weren't tutored in positive thinking.

Your outlook can affect your health and even lead to chronic mental illnesses like depression. I'll never forget a turning point in my own life. I was a student at Life Chiropractic College and working in the fitness room when a fellow student came in. We began talking about being positive through stressful times. I recall saying that from that time on I would make a conscious effort to not get too upset if a crisis hits. This commitment has made a huge difference in my life. I must remind myself of it daily, and, honestly, I find it quite difficult at times. I want to blow up and get angry when things happen, but even if I do, I replay in my mind that commitment I made many years ago, turn my thoughts around, and focus on good, not doom.

What I'm talking about is a conscious effort you must train on daily. Our most successful patients are the ones who accept where they are and strive for the best. They fight against the diagnosis the doctor may give them and won't accept the need for medication. With this fight comes action, action towards health, not a life of medication. If you accept the medication path, you lost the fight. It is easy to put a pill in your mouth and go on your merry way, but medication ALWAYS leads to other side effects in your body that aren't so merry after all. Damage always lies ahead. It takes a positive mind to believe you can have health without toxic waste being dumped through your blood stream. You can live a life without medication, but it first comes with an optimistic commitment to being drug free.

Posture and Your Mind

Standing tall or hunching over affects more than your appearance. It can change your outlook and brain chemistry. Psychologists call this "embodied cognition." Their research shows that how you move your muscles and where you place your limbs, head, and torso all help you control your mood, your behavior, and the way you think. Standing tall with good posture gives you a feeling of empowerment along with many other advantages. That is why chiropractors constantly encourage strong posture. It affects physical health, mental health, and our general outlook on life. Stand strong with shoulders back and head held high, and you will notice a difference in your physical and emotional health.

Even your facial expressions can have an effect. Research from Richard Petty, a psychologist and embodied cognition researcher at Ohio State University, shows that making a person put his face into the pose of a smile can lead him to happiness. "It's as if the happiness circuits go both ways," says Petty.

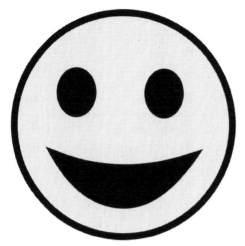

A smile, even a fake one, activates the feel-good regions of the brain. One recent study found that smiling even helped people's hearts return more quickly to a relaxed pace after exercise and other stresses, a sign of cardiac health. Psychologists say, "Neurons that fire together wire together." In other words, we spend so much time smiling when we're happy that eventually the smiling muscles parts of the brain get hooked up with the feel-good parts of the brain. This connection gets reinforced so many times that it doesn't even matter if you have a real reason to feel happy. Fake it and you'll make it. You actually re-wire your nerve system into a healthier response.

Stress

Get this straight: You will never have a stress-free life; therefore, you must learn how to properly respond to stress in order to make your immune system and body strong enough to withstand its effects. In other words, a strong immune system keeps your body from getting sick and breaking down.

The first thing that occurs when you are under stress is that your nervous system detects a stimulus that represents a physical threat or toxicity and/or deficiency, and then it must determine how to respond. For example, if you see a tiger chasing you, your body will make your leg muscles move extremely fast, your heart will work harder to pump blood to the muscles, your blood pressure will go up, your eyes will see where you need to run, and so on. These normal responses to the situation reflect the complete and amazing physiological response happening within your body without your having to think about it. Can you see why a healthy spine and nerve system are essential for health?

After you escape the tiger, or the eighteen wheeler that almost crashed into your car, or the unexpected visit from your mother-in-law, your body should go right back to normal physiological behavior. As your body relaxes, blood pressure will go down, sweating will stop, muscles will relax, and you will think clearly. You have responded normally; however, in today's hectic world, we put ourselves in stressful situations with work, projects that need to be completed by tomorrow, busy schedules, kids going to seven different sporting events all in one weekend, housework, yards to mow, and wives who are angry about it all! Living in such situations, the tiger at our heels every day and every hour, leads to physiological burnout. Blood pressure goes up and stays up, hormones will go down, hair begins to fall out, cortisol levels rise, belly fat increases, insomnia torments, anger comes easily, muscles tense, immune systems weaken, sickness comes every time someone sneezes, acid reflux kicks in, bowels stop moving regularly, hearts go out of rhythm, breathing problems, like asthma, begin, and we call it "aging"!

You cannot stay in a hectic environment without something giving in – your health, your heart, your marriage, your life! We call this a "sympathetic response" or a "fight or flight response." It's normal when being chased by a tiger, but a chronic state will lead to destruction and disease. Most Americans live there every day, and that is why we have so much sickness and disease. Your nerve system processes all of this stuff, and if your spine and nerve system are not functioning properly, the fight or flight response will be intensified because your body doesn't have the strength to battle. We'll cover more of this when our "ABC's" take us to "C," chiropractic.

This book will show you how to strengthen your body and immune system to control the effects of stress. Remember, stress will always be there, but now it doesn't have to drive you up the wall or into the grave.

Now, let's consider the medical approach to stress. When the effects of stress cause illness, what does the typical medical doctor do? Does he first look for the cause of the illness, or does he look for a drug to make you feel better? No brainer – he looks for the drug. If stress elevates your blood pressure, the doc finds a drug that may lower it without ever correcting the issue. This is dangerous because the physiological stress response is still running through your veins like caffeine from an espresso shot, but now you don't even feel it! Drugs hide the response and allow you to blindly continue down this destructive path. The doc may as well give you something to block the sensation of pain and then put your hand on a hot stove. "Stupid is as stupid does," Forrest. We do it every day in good ole America. Masking the pain is easier than changing your lifestyle, and it's a great money maker for pharmaceutical companies. And the beat goes on .....

Our Children

Sad to say, they're putting children on this medical hamster wheel at record rate. When I was a kid, not many students were on meds or lining up at the nurse's station to get a shot of inhaler, or taking boat loads of antidepressants, or being stamped as "ADHD." I knew a few who had to get allergy shots. I, too, acquired allergies but am completely healed of them now. Today, children on medication is "the new normal," and it's very disturbing. For various reasons – busyness, ignorance, etc. – parents don't investigate causes but simply "follow doctor's orders," go along with the crowd, and all of this equals pushing meds into their children.

If we continue to hold up drugs as the answer for every sickness and tummy ache, what will our kids turn to as they grow older? How will decades of medication eventually affect their health? Kids today can't even tolerate a skinned knee without some Ibuprofen. Do you blame the four-year-old or the parents who can't stand to hear him crying and have no fear of drug side effects?

We're raising wimps who depend on meds to block all discomfort. Well, guess what? Life does become uncomfortable sometimes, and if we don't learn to deal with it, we are in big trouble as we age. This applies to every aspect of life, not just our health.

Train a child in the way he should go, and when he is old he will not turn from it (Proverbs 22:6).

How are we training our kids to grow up? How are YOU training up your children? If your ATTITUDE is that they NEED a medication to get over every illness, fever, infection or cough, then you are training them to DEPEND on a drug for help at every bump in the road. That's a dangerous path to take.

Look at this growing trend:

- Eleven percent of school-age children are diagnosed with ADHD (attention deficit hyperactivity disorder), a twenty-two percent increase since 2003.

- One out of five boys is diagnosed with ADHD.

- About two-thirds of all children diagnosed with ADHD are prescribed medications that have dangerous side effects, and many are misdiagnosed.

- Fifty-four percent of children suffer from chronic illness such as obesity, asthma, and learning disabilities.

- Asthma currently affects over 7.1 million American children under age eighteen.

- Four million children and adolescents suffer from serious mental disorders.

- Suicide is the third leading cause of death in youth, ages fifteen to twenty-four.

- Antidepressant medication can increase suicidal thought and behavior in some children, adolescents, and young adults.

- Almost twenty-six percent of all US adults suffer from diabetes, one of the fastest growing diseases among children.

- One-third of all children, between ages two and nineteen, are overweight or obese. Most of these children will become diabetic.

- Childhood obesity has more than doubled with children and tripled with adolescents in the past thirty years.

- Obese youth are more likely to have risk factors for cardiovascular diseases such as high cholesterol or high blood pressure.

- Long-term effects of obesity increase the risk of diabetes, heart disease, stroke, and certain types of cancer.

- In 2009, the increase of prescription drug use among children was nearly four times higher than the overall population.

- One out of four insured children, and nearly thirty percent of adolescents, took at least one prescription medication to treat a chronic condition in 2009.

- American kids are the most medicated in the world, approximately three prescriptions per child, every year!

The Golden Pedestal

If you think that these statistics reflect some kind of normality and cannot be changed, then you're a victim of the system. If, however, you reject this so-called normality and decide that you and your children should not be sick, overweight, and over-medicated, then you're on the right track. Nothing more can be done if you play the role of the victim. Lie down and let the bus run over you. Not me! I'm a fighter who believes that we are born to greatness and our body can self-heal, through God's principles, and be strong and healthy without drugs. When YOU believe this way, you will continue to ask questions and demand logical answers. When you do demand answers from your medical doctor, he may throw you out of the office or simply tell you that YOU are NOT the doctor. Over the years, many, many of my patients have experienced such things simply because they wanted answers and human respect.

I view this arrogant "professional" attitude as the GOLDEN PEDESTAL! The doctor sees himself sitting high above the patient and above the general public, and you better not knock him off with your questions. Oh my – the high and mighty, but thank God I can say that I have personal friends, medical doctors who would never ever step onto that golden throne.

Your job is to question, not put people on pedestals. Listen, this is your body, your child – not theirs. It's your life, and you deserve answers and respect. We are all equal even though we have different educations and different jobs. Demand this equality from any doctor or practitioner you see.

I remember playing King of the Mountain as a kid. We would climb on to a dirt mound and try to keep the other kids from getting to the top. The goal was to push off any kid coming to the top. We wouldn't hurt each other but simply battled to hold our ground. Staying on top – you win! This reminds me of many doctors' attitudes. They will push you from asking questions and debating them. They will push you down and not allow you to succeed. I think it's a superiority thing, and they will feel weak if knocked down. Well, tough. This is your life and your health. One wrong medication or procedure could kill you or your kid or send you down a long road paved with drugs and a whole bunch of other problems. Don't go there! If a doctor, or any health practitioner, won't help you and work with you, go to another. There are plenty of doctors out there to choose from.

I like the verse in Matthew 11:25-26 where Jesus said, *I praise you, Father, Lord of Heaven and Earth, because you have hidden these things from the wise and learned, and revealed them to little children. Yes, Father, for this was Your good pleasure.* This reminds me of how simple but profound basic foundational health is – so simple that the educated cannot even see it. It sounds radical, crazy, and certainly not the norm at times. The children, however, do get it. When I talk to a child about health, it makes sense to him, but educated adults tend to over-analyze everything. They analyze their way right out of a simple solution because they believe things should be more complicated and "scientific."

B.J. Palmer, the developer of chiropractic, said, "It is so simple that it sounds crazy as hell. It is better to be crazy and have it work than to be educated and fail."

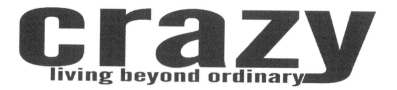

The attitude that the body is self-healing and self-regulating goes against the medical model. The medical model holds no place for a body that works through an illness without medication – a pill for a fever, a pill for a pain, a pill when you can't sleep, and a pill when you sleep too much – a pill for every ill.

What YOU Believe

What really matters here is what you believe or what you would like to believe. It may be a stretch of the imagination to picture yourself going a day without your medication or giving your kid a hug instead of a Tylenol, but what would you like to see happen? Would you like less or even NO medication? Can you picture yourself feeling amazingly well and not depending on ANY medication? How would you feel if your child didn't need those antibiotics or his ADHD or asthma drugs? How do you feel about the side effects of the meds you've been taking?

Change your ATTITUDE. Change your LIFE. Change your OUTCOME!

He who walks with the wise grows wise, but a companion of fools suffers harm (Proverbs 13:20).

This book, which you were smart enough to pick up because you value your life, provides wisdom that will transform and possibly save your life. You must start with the right attitude and then work on your health. Just because your friends, your family, your teachers, your neighbors, or even your pastor use medication like it's the best thing since sliced bread does not mean that it really is the best thing since sliced bread.

There is a way that seems right to a man, but in the end it leads to death (Proverbs 14:12).

When everyone else is running off to the doctor and taking meds with a victim mentality, buying into the diagnosis declared by their doctors, you need to question their beliefs, and, above all, question your own belief system. Take time to THINK and to PRAY.

A simple man believes anything, but a prudent man gives thought to his steps (Proverbs 14:15).

Test my information, and test the information from the medical community. Knowledge is power! The information I'm giving you is powerful, foundational, and simple – powerfully simple when you adhere to it. Test it out for yourself.

"An optimist is the one who sees a light where there is none. A pessimist is one who blows it out" (BJ Palmer).

Chapter 2

Behavior

Your behavior or your daily habits determine your future.

This section is NOT complicated; however, as Americans, this is where we tend to focus and where we encounter highly integrated marketing scams and gimmicks.

Jesus said, *If a blind man leads a blind man, both will fall into a pit (Matthew 15:14).*

When you get caught up in all the hype of the next diet pill, the newest discovery of some wild herb from Timbuktu, or some crazy combination of foods that will turn you into a twenty-year- old stud, you are going to be led away down a path with NO end in sight, a path built on shaky ground, a path far from the foundational principles of this book.

Behavior includes three basic things: what you eat, foundational supplements that compliment your nutrition, and how you move or exercise. That's it; so, let's jump right in.

Nutrition NOT Diet

Good nutrition is quite simple. Eat what God made, as much as possible, and eat processed food (man's food) as little as possible. It really could be that simple if we wouldn't get caught up in the latest and greatest but start with the foundation of nutrition and build from there. Nothing – no vitamin or exercise – can replace good, basic nutrition.

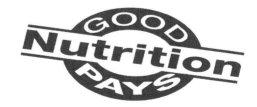

In Genesis it is written, *I give you every seed-bearing plant on the face of the earth and every tree that has fruit with seed in it. They will be yours for food.* This has not changed over the years. We must eat this way daily.

Listen to the words of Dr. Palmer, written and interpreted by Dr. Stephenson in his chiropractic textbook: "Poison is any substance introduced into, or manufactured within the living body, upon which Innate Intelligence, after becoming cognizant of its presence through the interpretation of the vibrations set up in the tissue cells, and knowing that such a substance cannot be utilized, and if allowed to remain in the body will be absorbed by the tissue cells and do damage, begins a systematic process of elimination from the body." WOW!

Any substance introduced into or manufactured within the living body, which Innate Intelligence cannot use in metabolism, is a poison. Medicine is a poison because it is a substance that Innate Intelligence does not prepare for use in the body. Medicine is a substance given to "stimulate" or "inhibit" body function.

Food can also be a poison to the body. Anything made or prepared artificially and then introduced into the body, against which Innate Intelligence rebels, is a poison. Modern man creates many foods altered from their original design by God. This alteration affects their digestive ability in the body, thus making them a poison to our body. Too much food creates an imbalance and will add stress to the body, which can likewise lead to dis-ease. Too little food creates an imbalance and also will add stress to the body, which can lead to dis-ease. This also applies to the nutritional content. If you are eating processed, low nutrient-dense food, you will also create an imbalance over time, which creates dis-ease in the cells and organs, which then leads to dysfunction.

Dis-ease is when the body is out of ease. In the early stages of dysfunction, you will not even feel the effects of this stress in your body. Early stages of arteries clogging, early stages of

32

cancer cells attacking your breast or prostate, early stages of Alzheimer's, or even early stages of kidney stones developing, all begin with the body dropping out of "ease" and beginning the disease process. You will not feel or notice the effect until it has reached a breaking point.

The food you eat and your daily habits create balance, health and vitality or slowly pull your body away from balance and lead to dis-ease and dysfunction.

Your Innate Intelligence

When your body is so far away from balance, you desperately attempt to "diet" your way back to health. Dieting, a poor approach to health, attempts to regulate or alter/shock your body into submission. Diet pills, diets, surgery, or starving yourself, just like the medical approach, all do something contrary to the wisdom of your Innate Intelligence. Forcing your body to change with chemicals is the absolutely ridiculous approach that got you into this situation to begin with. Poor choices, poor nutrition, chemicals in your food, overeating and lack of good nutrients are the very reasons most Americans end up obese or overweight.

We, thank God, have found a way, through good nutrients, proper nutrition, and pure water, to assist in getting your body back on track. Once there, you should have no problem staying fit and healthy if you apply the basic principles in this book.

Your Innate Intelligence knows exactly what your body needs and how to utilize the proper nutrients for repair, regeneration and healing. You do your job by supplying your body with good nutrition. Your Intelligence will take over the minute you put the food in your mouth and belly. If you give your body the wrong food, your Intelligence will do the very best in the situation, but will fall short every time. In fact, when you do not supply your body with the right nutrients, your Innate Intelligence will extract the necessary nutrients and elements from other tissue to make the proper chemical changes needed for energy, digestion, or repair, thus creating more weaknesses in your body. Soon enough, you will start to feel the effects.

Food Choices Made Simple:

1. Fresh fruit
   a. Best if organic, without chemicals
   b. Best if fresh
   c. Frozen berries and fruit for shakes or cold snacks
   d. Great for every meal, snacks, and handy to carry with you wherever you go
   e. Best if eaten first, before your other food
   f. Can be eaten as much as you desire

2. Fresh vegetables
   a. Best if organic
   b. Best if fresh or frozen
   c. Great at every meal, for fresh veggie snacks, and in ziploc bags when you're on the go
   d. Best if eaten first, along with fruit
   e. Large salad, once or twice a day
   f. A better choice than fries when eating out
   g. Flavor tremendously enhanced with olive oil and sea salt

3. Lean protein
   a. Beef, turkey, fish, eggs, chicken
   b. Wild game always a great choice
   c. Wild, not farm-raised fish
   d. Organic, free-range, no hormones, and no steroids
   e. Not overcooked or charred when grilling
   f. To be eaten at every meal, the size of your palm
   g. Excess fat trimmed
   h. Should be eaten slowly and chewed thoroughly

4. Fats
    a. Extra virgin olive oil, coconut oil, butter (preferably raw/organic)
    b. Raw nuts and seeds
    c. Avocado
    d. Almond butter or other organic butters (peanut has mold)

5. Water and Juice
    a. Clean, pure, alkaline, distilled or spring water – not tap water
    b. As much as desired – if thirsty you are already dehydrated
    c. Best to drink water slowly, all day long
    d. Fresh vegetable juice a great choice
    e. Limit fresh fruit juice to one glass daily if needed
    f. Limited amount of processed juice – too much sugar and calories
    g. Limit to 2-3 cups of coffee per day if needed
    h. Must eliminate: soda, monster drinks, other energy drinks, diet drinks (and anything diet – dangerous chemicals)
6. Grains
    a. Must be whole grain, 100% grain or sprouted
    b. Limited to one serving per day
    c. Not necessary for health
    d. Use sparingly!

That's a basic outline. I know there are a million and one diets and combinations of how to eat, times to eat, highest nutrient-dense foods, highest chemicals, etc. You must, however, lock and load the basics first before trying other fancy approaches. I am giving you the foundation – simple and powerful!

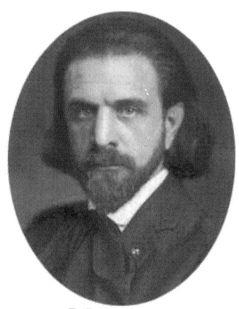

B.J. PALMER
DEVELOPER OF CHIROPRACTIC

"While other professions are concerned with changing environment to suit the weakened body, Chiropractic is concerned with strengthening the body to 'suit' the environment" (B.J. Palmer).

The foods you eat support the amazing Intelligence in your body to do exactly what it needs for repair and healing. You don't have to stimulate or inhibit, but you do need to remove interference and allow the Intelligence of your body to do its thing. Innate Intelligence expresses itself through your body, and your food can add to this expression or destroy it. Your Intelligence wants and desires health and will do everything it can to defend against your poor choices and the lack of nutrients supplied. Support your body with good food choices!

When you sit to dine with a ruler, note well what is before you, and put a knife to your throat if you are given to gluttony. Do not crave his delicacies, for that food is deceptive (Proverbs 23; 1-3).

Those are strong, Biblical words – not mine; so, listen to this advice and stay away from the delicacies (sweets, donuts, Danish pastries, candy, ice cream) as much as possible, especially if they are leading to obesity or gluttony.

Interesting research by Dr. James Chestnut, from his book, *The Innate Diet and Natural Hygiene*:

- Some evidence shows that what we eat changes the expression of our genes.

- A Purdue University study has showed that kids low in omega-3 essential fatty acids are significantly more likely to be hyperactive, have learning disorders, and to display behavioral problems.

- The modern diet is dangerously deficient in omega-3 and gamma omega-6 fatty acids.

- The modern diet is dangerously toxic with unhealthy forms of omega-6 linoleic fatty acids.

- The human brain is more than 60% structural fat, which depends on healthy levels of omega-3 fatty acids.

- The pH level of our internal fluids affects every cell in our bodies. The entire metabolic process depends on an alkaline environment.

- Insulin levels affect the immune system. High insulin levels stimulate the sympathetic nervous system which in turn causes an increase in stress hormones like cortisol which inhibit the cell-mediated immune system.

- One saltine cracker will cause the blood sugar to go over 100, and in many people it will cause the blood sugar to go to 150.

- Eating sugar decreases your immune system.

- Insulin is involved in the storage of magnesium. One major role for magnesium is to relax muscles. When you lose magnesium and your smooth muscles in your blood vessels relax, your blood vessels constrict, leading to a chronic increase in blood pressure! But listen, the answer is not to take magnesium. The answer is to eat less sugar!

- Insulin is termed a mytogenic hormone, which means it stimulates cell proliferation or cell division. This can lead to chronic sickness, disease, and even cancer.

- A high carbohydrate diet produces a lot of insulin to decrease blood sugar. You end up with low blood sugar so your body produces cortisol to level it out. Cortisol increases belly fat and also produces catecholamines, which makes you nervous and stimulates your brain to crave carbohydrates and fat!

- This stress also eats up your serotonin levels, thereby leading to depression!

Weight Loss

With the number of obese and overweight Americans skyrocketing, we need to address this issue. Being overweight or obese is unnatural to the body and unhealthy. The stress it puts on your body increases every illness and will lead to chronic health problems. Poor behavior and poor choices, not genetics or bad luck, create obesity; so, better behavior and better choices will lead to health and long-term energy and strength.

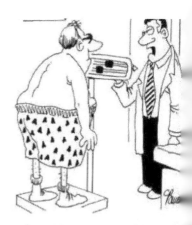

"No, it's not water. You seem be retaining food."

Eating unhealthy goes way beyond looking fat or frumpy. It affects your nervous system, brain function, immune system, and every cell in your body. Most weight loss programs out there, however, do not address the complete picture. That's why I never wanted to get involved in weight loss. There are too many weight loss gurus out there, too many stupid programs that have a bad name to them, but I saw weight loss as a necessity to help my patients get healthy. As you will learn in the next chapter on chiropractic, our spine and nerve system comprise the most amazing and most important system of our body; however, even with a healthy and strong nervous system, if we eat unhealthy or have poor habits, we will never achieve optimal health. Likewise, if we eat extremely healthy and exercise without a properly functioning nerve system, we will never achieve optimal health.

When I began to investigate the weight loss programs out there, I found several things:

1. Participants take six to twelve months to lose twenty pounds, at best.

2. The average cost to lose twenty pounds is over $3,300.

3. Programs sell boxed food, which is far from healthy.

4. Programs demand intense exercise for up to one hour per day.

5. The regimens do not reset the body's internal healing power and metabolism.

6. The gurus focus on one piece of the puzzle, such as food.

7. Many programs require dangerous drugs.

8. The more radical programs require extremely dangerous surgery.
9. Most people on these programs gain their weight back because they don't identify the underlying cause of the problem.

10. Many people who lose weight don't feel healthy.

11. Most people depend on supplements, drugs, boxed food, or some crazy diet to keep the weight off.

My interest in weight loss developed out of my own need. You see, as my patients were asking how to lose weight, my answer was always the same – eat better and exercise more, but my advice never seemed to work, not even for me. After I turned forty, within just five years, I had gained ten pounds and two inches on my waist. I couldn't figure how this was happening to me. I have always exercised, run marathons and ultra-marathons, entered competitive 5K races, lifted weights, and ate healthy. My quest for the answer involved several difference programs that restricted me and resulted in overnight weight gain if I messed up. I heard of one crazy program that suggested taking an ice bath to shiver and somehow burn off extra calories. Thank God I had the sense to avoid that one!

I finally found the right program and lost ten pounds in ten days and two inches off my waist in twenty days. The youthful feeling this easy to implement program gave me proved that I had reset my body and convinced me to present it to my staff, family, and patients. We have refined this very successful program over the years and employed the proper testing to get amazing results in every patient.

The program's key components:

1. Cleansing, detoxification, and purification of the body: You must understand that toxins based on diet, environment, medications, and even tap water fill your body on a daily basis. You counteract these things by supplying your body with the proper nutrients so your Innate Intelligence can begin to repair and heal at a cellular level.

2. The program enables you to boost your hormone levels without dangerous synthetic medication or even bio-identical hormones, which can lead to a big expense and a lot of testing.

3. The burning of abnormal body fat: I'm not talking about muscle, water, or organ fat. I'm talking about belly and booty fat, the abnormal fat, which is stored energy, ready to be used. Your body just needs to tap into that.

4. Increased alkalinity and restored hydration: This means pure alkaline water and healthy food choices, which you can buy at any store. You can utilize other supplements when necessary, depending on age, health history, medication and your ultimate goal.

5. The main goal for all weight loss patients in the program is not just to lose weight but also to get healthy! We can be skinny and sick. We can be athletic and have cancer or heart disease. Losing weight does not make you healthy. Losing weight properly and identifying the underlying cause of weight gain and correcting it will make you healthy. This sets us apart from every other program out there. Chronic sickness and obesity come from long-term poor habits. Long-term health comes from healthy habits and a healthy nerve system.

6. Focus on the nerve system: As you will learn, the nerve system controls every function of your body. Your brain and nerve system digest your food, stimulate and balance your hormone activity, control thyroid output, evacuate or eliminate waste through peristalsis, control the proper acid balance in your stomach, keep your bones of normal density, and help balance brain function to maintain health. Your ability to lose weight and be healthy starts in the brain and nerve system. We test for this and it is usually a major part in losing weight and keeping it off.

Key Factors in Total Health

As you can see from these key components, unless you focus on complete health, you will fall far short. Stephenson's *Chiropractic Textbook* emphasizes significant factors involved in this total health:

1. The Poisons of Environment

    a) Abnormal or extremely adverse environmental conditions for the human body are important in the study of the cause of dis-ease. They affect the health by making normal adaptation more difficult if not impossible. They are not considered the cause of dis-ease, or even secondary causes, but they further enhance the limitations of matter.

    b) If subluxations exist, and in most people they do, especially those affecting the elimination organs, the effect is still worse.

    c) Some environmental conditions, such as unsanitary surroundings, will poison even a healthy person.

    d) The possibilities of environmental poisoning include: impure water, air, food, bad climate, poor sanitation, poor hygiene, personal and environmental, effluvia and germs.

2. Water as an Environmental Factor

    a) Water may poison a body of lowered resistance when it is impure, impregnated with injurious minerals, stagnant, charged with poisonous gases, etc.

    b) Pure water for human consumption contains none of these but may have harmless and normal amounts of minerals and germs.

c) Innate Intelligence warns the educated mind by smell, taste, and sight, and depends upon educational adaptation for safety.

3. Food as an Environmental Factor

   a) Abnormal food may poison a body of lowered resistance when it is impure or contains impurities such as poisonous chemicals and poisonous gases or if it has changed chemically, decomposed, etc.

   b) Pure food for human consumption must be free from any of these impurities.

Our body needs purity. Any foreign item, chemical, or poison to the body is harmful. Quite simply, the Innate Intelligence in your body is always trying to maintain balance and health. Stated as Chiropractic Principle #21, the mission of Innate Intelligence is to maintain the material of the body of a "living thing" in active organization. Our Innate Intelligence will take what we give it in order to organize cellular repair and healing. That is why supplying healthy food, water and environmental factors, free of toxins and poison, are essential for healing and health.

Your Innate Intelligence is fighting an uphill battle if you continue to give it sugar, processed food, toxic water, soda, bad fats, and poor nutrition. It will do its best, but your body will eventually break down and develop dis-ease. It is quite amazing that we live past five or six with such a horrible diet and very little nutrition. We abuse our body and still survive. The question is, do you want to thrive or merely survive?

Regarding nutrition, consider Chiropractic Principle #24: The Limits of Adaptation. This principle states that Innate Intelligence adapts forces and matter for the body as long as it can do so without breaking a universal law, or Innate Intelligence as limited by the limitations of matter. In other words, we are limited by what we supply our body. If you continue to abuse your body, there are limitations to the amount of healing your body will have; thus, chronic sickness and disease sets in. Your extremely intelligent brain wants not only to function properly but to function at the highest level. How you treat your body will manifest in health or sickness.

Do you not know that your body is a temple of the Holy Spirit, who is in you, whom you have received from God? You are not your own; you were bought at a price. Therefore honor God with your body (1 Corinthians 6:19-20).

Do you treat your body as a temple? How about a wooden shack? This is your body and your life. How you treat your body has an outcome, which brings us to Chiropractic Principle #17, Cause and Effect. Every effect has a cause, and every cause has effects. The study of Chiropractic is largely a study of the relations between cause and effect, and effect and cause. Let this sink in. Every choice you make has an effect on your body and life. Compare eating an apple to eating a donut. One choice adds life; one adds destruction. Sitting on your couch and watching another boring television show or going for a walk or jog – both have an effect on your body, negative or positive.

Supplements

There are thousands of vitamins, herbs, homeopathic remedies, and other natural supplements to choose from. So where do you start?

I remember when I was first in practice and I wanted to really understand how to help my patients the best I could. Then one day, a vitamin salesman came into my office. His natural supplemental concoction sounded wonderful. This vitamin cure-all had me totally hooked. My quest for finding the best vitamins began, a quest full of books, seminars, and every different kind of supplement that seemed right for my family and me.

I was starting to depend on something I could put into my mouth instead of what was truly necessary and essential. This vitamin cure seemed to be a big part of the health puzzle. Not so! I eventually realized that we must eat healthy food first and take vitamins, herbs, or homeopathic remedies for short-term use at best. Incessant consumption of supplements merely offers a different form of "treatment," and that is not what my practice is all about. Am I any better than a medical doctor if I simply substitute a bag of vitamins for a bunch of drugs and poisons?

The plethora of vitamins and herbs totally confused me. I didn't want to play that game. How on earth could I even guess what you really need? Only your God-given Innate Intelligence would know; so, I reversed my approach to supplements and now only carry a minimal amount in my office. I believe we have a few essential nutrients that can support our body, brain, nerve system, and immune system, designed as part of our daily intake of food and lifestyle but not optimally available in our food supply. Let's take a look them.

1. Fish Oil

It is well known that the modern diet is dangerously deficient in omega-3 fatty acids and overboard in unhealthy omega-6 fatty acids. The ideal fatty acid ratio should range from 2:1 to 1:1, omega-6: omega-3. Experts estimate a ratio between 15:1 and 22:1 in the standard American diet.

With grass-fed meat, healthy fish, and healthy oils such olive and coconut oil in our daily consumption, we would not need to supplement. Because our cattle and other livestock are grain and corn-fed and our fish are farm-raised, we do not get the healthy fats from either source. In fact, we continue to eat fried food and hydrogenated oils throughout the day, thereby putting the ratio way out of balance.
The human brain is more that 60% structural fat and depends on healthy fats. A lack of omega-3 fatty acids will affect your thinking, mood, hormones, energy, behavior, and much more.

Your brain, the main fuse box in your "house," must optimally function in order for the other parts of your body to optimally perform. This explains why omega-3 deficiencies can be tied to dyslexia, violence, depression, memory problems, weight gain, cancer, heart disease, eczema, allergies, inflammatory diseases, arthritis, and diabetes. Many studies on depression show that omega-3 fatty acids, along with exercise, yield far better results than the antidepressant medications.

The most important thing is to add healthy fats to your diet and remove all those fried foods and hydrogenated and partially hydrogenated oils out of your diet. Unsure? Read the labels! Regarding supplements, a minimum of two capsules or 2,000 mgs per day is best. When fighting inflammation from injury, trauma or stress, as high as 6,000 – 10,000 mgs per day may be necessary. Again, to try to exactly understand what your body needs is impossible. Training for marathons, I used to have a long run of fifteen to eighteen miles. I soon discovered my joints, especially my knees, would hurt and swell for the following one to three days; so I tried taking eight fish oil capsules the day before I ran and two days following. The results were fantastic: NO pain or swelling! Fish oil is a great anti-inflammatory; however, you MUST buy high quality oil because many are rancid or full of toxins such as mercury.

2. Vitamin D

A significant relationship exists between vitamin D levels and immune function, including chronic colds, seasonal flu, heart disease, and even cancer. Low vitamin D levels put you at higher risk for chronic sickness and disease. The research noted by Dr. James Chestnut states that vitamin D up-regulates the genetic expression of AMPs (antimicrobial peptides) in immune cells. Along with that, vitamin D plays an important role in controlling the inflammatory response initiated by specialized immune cells called macrophages. A deficiency of vitamin D means deficient control of inflammation. In the skin, vitamin D also activates the immune system against antigens.

Sunlight is the best source of vitamin D. You only need bare skin exposure for fifteen minutes per day; however, with busy work schedules and during the winter months, especially in the north (and even more so in Pittsburgh), it is hard to get even that fifteen minutes. Your second best source is cod liver oil, but it must be pure and free of toxins. I have always loved the sun and still love to play with the kids outside in the summertime. My dark tan as a kid convinced me that I was part Indian. All summer long, then and now, I've enjoyed the sunshine without all those harmful, toxic suntan lotions. You cannot convince me that sunlight causes cancer. It's a senseless argument. If God is light, how could light be bad, and why would He create something that causes cancer? I believe that the toxic medications raging through our bodies, including our skin, chemically react with the sun and the poisonous lotions. Remember Chemistry class? Put some chemicals in a glass test tube under a Bunsen burner, and watch it boil over or explode. Do you think this could happen when the heat of the sun interacts with all the chemicals in your body? I do!

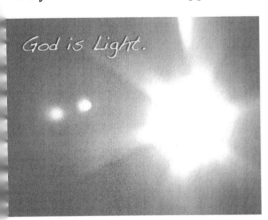

God is Light.

This is the message we have heard from Him and announce to you, that God is light, and in Him there is no darkness at all (1 John 1:5).

Every good and perfect gift is from above, coming down from the Father of the heavenly lights, who does not change like shifting shadows" (James 1:17).
For the LORD God is a sun and shield; the LORD bestows favor and honor; no good thing does he withhold from those whose walk is blameless (Psalm 84:11).

The LORD is my light and my salvation; whom shall I fear? The LORD is the stronghold of my life – of whom shall I be afraid (Psalm 27:1)?

And God said, "Let there be light," and there was light (Genesis 1:3).

I often thought that if God created light and God resembles light, could that be why we are so attracted to light, to the very source that created us? With God radiating into our soul and being, wouldn't that create a sense of spiritual uplifting and a positive mental attitude? Should you be afraid of light? Sunlight causing cancer? I would suggest not to get burned and not to cause damage to your skin. Be sensible, and try to get your fifteen minutes per day. It will change your mood and give your body energy. My patients always have a healthier smile and attitude on a bright and sunny day here in Pittsburgh. Sunlight is good. Vitamin D is good.

3. **Probiotics**

Probiotics are health-promoting bacteria required for proper digestion of food and immune defense against illnesses promoting bacteria, viruses, and fungi. The human body contains 90% microorganisms and only 10% human cells. We consume far below what we need to maintain the healthy levels of good bacteria. Research shows that we now consume one millionth of the healthy probiotic bacteria that we did before pesticides, herbicides, and industrial farming became commonplace.

Good bacteria are essential for healing, fighting against infections, and raising your immune system for defense. Without a healthy immune system and good bacteria, you are left with very little fighting power. No wonder so many people get sick and chronically sick. We used to get a normal amount of good bacteria from fresh fruits and vegetables grown in healthy soil, especially when ingested raw; however, with extreme spraying and over-production of crops on the same soil, thus depleting its nutrients , plus all the commercial foods we consume, our bodies are void of good bacteria. On top of all that, we destroy whatever good bacteria is left by overdosing on doctor-prescribed antibiotics and the antibiotics in the animals whose meat we buy from the grocery store.

Without an army of good bacteria to defend us, our immune systems are compromised and our bodies made vulnerable to many health disorders such as the following:

- Diarrhea
- Digestive disorders
- Immune deficiency
- Fibromyalgia
- Asthma
- Heart disease
- Cancer
- Infections (ear, bladder, bronchial, sinus)

All of these lead to decreased health and vitality. This is especially important if you have taken antibiotics in the past (especially within the past year); eaten non-organic meat, processed foods (sugar, grains, white flour products), or dairy; have made other poor lifestyle choices.

Supplements are meant to support your system, not fix it. You cannot take supplements to create health if your diet and lifestyle are broken; however, if your diet and lifestyle are not in order, supplementing with fish oil, vitamin D, and probiotics can keep you afloat – a simple and affordable way to support your health before chronic sickness and dis-ease strike. You'll find it much cheaper and easier to prevent disease rather than manage it!

I have seen this in my own life and love this simple approach. I find it a lot easier to eat a healthy diet and take a few supplements rather than trying to balance all my nutritional needs through vitamins and herbs. The question is: where do we begin? Well, if you like simple and if you like powerful, I have a plan for YOU! You need to think like a child, don't overcomplicate things, and "keep it simple, stupid" – KISS!

He called a little child and had him stand among them. And he said: "I tell you the truth, unless you change and become like little children, you will never enter the kingdom of heaven. Therefore, whoever humbles himself like this child is the greatest in the kingdom of heaven (Matthew 18:2-4).

I understand what Jesus is saying in this verse, and if we apply the inherent principle to our health, things become easy. Think like a child , and do some simple, yet profound, things. A little child, before being taught otherwise, would choose a brightly colored orange over some dull, ugly processed fries. Childlike. Choose wisely, and it will keep you alive!

Take the 90-day challenge. Take your fish oil, vitamin D, and probiotics daily and see what happens. Several months ago, I had an infected tooth. Antibiotics were prescribed, and I was told that my tooth needed to be pulled. A second opinion offered the same advice. This was after my two-week African safari during which I did not have access to my supplements. Instead of the antibiotics, I took four probiotic pills, eight fish oils, and vitamin D drops. By the end of the day – no pain! I was able to get by for ten days before getting the tooth pulled.

Exercise

In my previous book, I took a much deeper view of this. This time, let's do it simple and easy. Exercise is critical for optimal neurological development, physical strength, chemical balance, hormonal success, and just a good strong body to keep you upright and walking until the day you leave this earth. You don't want to meet your Maker crippled up in a wheelchair. To go out with a high hand, you must exercise, move, and be active for life.

I often ask people this question: "What is the best exercise?" I seldom get the correct answer, which is - THE ONE YOU LIKE TO DO AND WILL DO FOR LIFE. Sure, there are some exercises that are better for long-term health, joint health, and posture, but if you don't do them, nothing happens.

I enjoy lifting weights and running as my two staples to health. I tried other things, but this is what works for me. I love to play sports and compete; so, being in shape and strong makes me competitive at a ripe young age of forty-seven. I believe that you must do both cardiovascular exercise, or aerobic type exercise, AND weight training, or resistance training, to be your best. Find your two forms of exercise and begin. Action is key!

First, let's look at some research from Dr. James Chestnut's book, *Innate Physical Fitness and Spinal Hygiene.* Consider his points regarding how exercise affects your genes:

- Exercise induces normal expression of your genome (your hereditary information).

- Physical inactivity produces an abnormal gene expression and is a direct causal factor of most chronic health conditions by its direct alteration of gene expression.
- Your genes are programmed to express health, but your lifestyle and the environment you live in program them.

- Genes are like a library. You inherit your books from your parents, but you inherit healthy books 99.9% of the time. Less than 0.1% of health problems in society are classified as genetic disorders.

- It is impossible to be well without providing the innate genetic intelligence with exercise and good posture.

Approximately 70% of adults in the United States do not undertake the recommended thirty minutes of moderate physical activity five or more times per week, which includes those 24% of Americans who have no physical activity. A Scandinavian twin study showed that 58 – 100% of site-specific cancers had an environmental origin. The Harvard Center for Cancer Prevention in a 1996 report estimated that, of the total number of cancer deaths, 30% were due to tobacco, 30% to adult diet and obesity, 5% to occupational factors, and 2% to environmental pollution. This report predated much of the work regarding exercise's preventive effect on many site-specific cancers. A total of 91% of the cases of Type 2 diabetes and 82% of the coronary artery disease cases in 84,000 female nurses could be attributed to habits and so-called high-risk behavior [defined in the study as body mass index (BMI) greater than twenty-five, diet low in cereal fibers and polyunsaturated fat and high in transfat and glycemic load, a sedentary lifestyle, and currently smoking].

Physical inactivity is the third leading cause of death in the United States and contributes to the second leading cause (obesity), accounting for at least one in ten deaths. Aerobic exercise elevates blood levels of high density cholesterol, lowers blood pressure and resting heart rate, decreases platelet aggregability as well as the tendency for vasoconstriction, and enhances endothelial health as determined by post-ischemic brachial artery vasodialation. In layman's terms, exercise cleanses and heals your blood and cardiovascular system.

A very important benefit of resistance exercise (weight training) and other maximal effort exercise patterns is that they raise heart rates very high. This is proving to be important for heart health and homeostasis (a state of stability) as this is what our genes expect. Simply jogging or walking does not elicit this heart rate variability and challenge, which is so necessary for heart health. In other words, you must push yourself with high intensity exercise such as sprinting or going as fast as you can for twenty to thirty seconds during your training session.

Exercise also increases antioxidants. Antioxidants are substances such as vitamin C, vitamin E, and beta carotene which protect the body's cells from oxidation. (To make it simple, think of oxidation as a process that makes your body rust out.) You can spend a ton of money on antioxidant supplements, which can be beneficial; however, never dismiss the role of good old-fashioned exercise.

Physical inactivity, as shown in sixty-one studies involving 2,200 subjects, decreased blood HDL cholesterol by 4.4%, which would be an approximate reduction in risk for coronary heart disease by 4% in men and 6% in women. You could take debilitating cholesterol drugs or search the grocery store shelves for foods touted as "low cholesterol," or you could simply eat a healthy diet, as we discussed earlier, and get your body moving.

Sedentary men and women had a 56% and 72%, respectively, higher incidence of melanomas than those exercising five to seven days a week. Exercising four days or less per week provided no protection from melanomas. You gotta' make it a part of your daily life. BE ACTIVE! Remember Sir Isaac Newton? No, he wasn't a British rock star from the 70's. He was a brilliant scientist born in the 1600's who discovered the "laws of motion."

You might not remember studying him in school, but regarding the topic of exercise, please remember one thing that he found out: A BODY IN MOTION TENDS TO STAY IN MOTION UNLESS ACTED ON BY AN OUTSIDE FORCE. Keep moving! And don't YOU be one of the "outside forces" that hinders your own movement!

Chapter 3

Chiropractic

I believe I have saved the best for last. In the ABC's of Health, C – Chiropractic – is the electricity behind the scenes. It is the intelligence, the artist, the creator, and the developer, which coordinates all the beauty on how you express life. As you read, take time to visualize this amazing process and intelligence, and you will begin to appreciate how God so magnificently created you and why your nerve system is the Master System. My attempt to capture this most amazing intelligence and explain how this master system works will be my best attempt. I don't believe we can fathom the depths of God's intelligence in our human body and all its intricacies, but here goes...

Let's set the stage for this chiropractic section. You have to realize that describing how God designed the body and just how everything works so miraculously is quite a task. Describing the intricacies of cellular function, neurological connection, repair, development, hormonal balance, along with all the other components of our body, is overwhelming.

For You created my inmost being; you knit me together in my mother's womb. I praise You because I am fearfully and wonderfully made; Your works are wonderful, I know that full well. My frame was not hidden from You when I was made in the secret place. When I was woven together in the depths of the earth, Your eyes saw my unformed body" (Psalm 139: 13-16a).

Take a silent moment sometime today to just look in the mirror at your beauty – your hair that crowns your head, eyebrows perfectly positioned over your eyes designed to see a glorious sunset, your fingers formed to meticulously thread a needle, legs to carry you to a mountaintop, arms to lift your child, and lips to kiss his cheek. On and on it goes. As you take a moment to visualize how each part of your body works and how and why it was designed the way it was, it is quite breathtaking. Deepen your understanding of this by reading *In the Likeness of God* by Philip Yancey and Dr. Paul Brand.

But the things that come out of a person's mouth come from the heart, and these defile them (Matthew 15:18),

Above all else, guard your heart, for everything you do flows from it (Proverbs 4:23).

How does your body express itself? Just like Godliness is the expression of your spiritual life, your physical health is the expression of how your nerve system functions. What comes out of your mouth is directly related to what is stored up in your heart. How your organs, glands, muscles, and hormones work is directly related to the nerve supply coming from your brain through the spinal cord and out of the nerve. Your nerve system directly controls just how your body functions.

If you are reading your Bible daily, memorizing verses, trusting in God, going to church, praying daily, meditating, and listening to Christian radio, then what comes out of your mouth is Godliness and holiness. You are thankful, and your attitude will reflect true spiritual health. Likewise, if your nerve system is 100% connected to every cell, muscle, and organ (your stomach, heart, colon, lungs, spleen, arms and legs, shoulders, etc.), then your physical body will express health. The stomach will not have acid reflux, the lungs will be free from infection or asthma, your heart will beat in perfect rhythm, your bowels will eliminate waste daily, your arms and legs will be without numbness/tingling or pain, and every organ, cell and muscle will work properly. You will express physical health. Your nerve system will deliver your level of health.

Very Important: Your nerve system is your Master system which controls and coordinates all other organs/parts of your body. You CANNOT be at your optimal health if your nerve system cannot carry the mental impulses from your brain to your body parts! We are fearfully and wonderfully designed, and this amazing creation and physical body is directly run by your nerve system. Think of how a baby is created in the mother's womb. Each day, week and month, a new part of the body develops. Cells begin to connect and build the heart, eyes, liver, etc. The nerve system builds each part! After birth, each part is run by the nerve system. This creates repair from injury, an immune system to fight infection, bone development to rebuild a broken bone, and digestion of a simple carrot to strengthen your eyes. If you actually take a few minutes to really fathom this great, amazing process, you'll find it quite overwhelming and hard to find words to describe the beauty of it all.

If your nerve system created and organized the perfect development of your body, and if your nerve system directly controls your health and daily repairs every organ, gland, cell, and muscle, shouldn't you take this nerve system thing seriously? After reading this section, you will get a whole new perspective and appreciation for your spine and nerve system. You will get a deeper understanding why we as chiropractors adjust the spine and keep movement, balance, and alignment in the spine. You'll know why we must look to the nerve system first and coordinate the highest neurological connection before we alter the body with chemicals or surgically remove its parts. You will receive a newfound hope that you can return to health and that your body does have the ability to heal. You will understand the principles of healing. You will be able to EXPRESS health as never before IF you ACT upon this information!

Therefore everyone who hears these words of mine and puts them into practice is like a wise man who built his house on the rock (Matthew 7:24). If you merely listen to the words of Jesus and fail to act upon them, your foundation will be weak. You must act.

Where there are no oxen, the manger is empty, but from the strength of an ox comes an abundant harvest (Proverbs 14:4). This means that there is no milk without some manure. Some disturbance or work is the price of growth and accomplishment. You cannot attain health without work and action!

As you begin to understand chiropractic, you will no longer ask, "Does that stuff really work?" To the contrary, your thinking will become more logical and urgent, and you'll want to know, "Where is the nearest chiropractor who can help me analyze my spine and my health, remove subluxations, and keep me aligned for the rest of my life, and does he have a workable plan to include my other family members?"

As you begin to understand chiropractic, you will realize that healing at your highest level and reaching

Do you know anyone who would like:

60% less hospital admissions
59% less days in the hospital
62% less outpatient surgeries
85% less in pharmaceutical costs

A 7-year study showed that patients whose primary physician was a chiropractor, experienced the above results.

For the health of your loved ones...

CHOOSE CHIROPRACTIC

Journal of Manipulative and Physiological Therapy, May 2007; 30(4): 263-269, Richard L. Sarnat, MD, James Winterstein, DC, Jerilyn A. Cambron, DC, PhD

your ultimate health potential cannot be achieved if your spine is out of alignment and there is stress on your nerves, no matter how well you eat, how much time you spend at the gym, or how strong your genetic makeup is. Chiropractic care is about optimizing your nerve system and all about neurology – not pain, headaches, or any other symptom. Your understanding will enable you to see how your body will heal from those conditions when it FUNCTIONS properly. For example, you don't eat food to heal your asthma; you eat food to survive. You don't get adjusted to heal your asthma; you get adjusted to allow your body to function optimally at 100% nerve energy, thus setting your body up for optimal healing. Asthma conditions will resolve themselves when your body functions properly and you practice healthy lifestyle habits. Then, after you get into alignment and your body heals itself, you can continue to enjoy optimal health and life as you continue with regular spinal adjustments and the healthy habits that allowed your body to heal in the first place.

If we, as parents, start these healthy habits and lifestyle choices for our children at their birth, they will avoid the health problems that plague so many adults. It sure is a lot easier and a lot more fun to simply maintain your health, and the health of your kids, than it is to fight to get it back after years of pain and suffering.

Where It Begins

When conception begins, the sperm and egg join to start to create life. Two cells divide to become four, then eight, sixteen, and so on. Within a week, over a hundred cells are created into a ball. Cells will continue to divide and create seventy-five trillion cells that make up a human body. WOW!

The FIRST things to develop are the brain, spinal cord and nerves – the system that coordinates the makeup of your body, like the branches of a tree that yields its fruit. The brain is your center hub or master control system, which sends information through the spinal cord and out of the nerves to create your heart, face, arms, legs, sex organs, and muscles.

So, what would you guess to be the most important system of your body? The very system that created the development of ALL of your organs – your nervous system, the most amazing system you have, not only to create life, but to sustain life for one hundred twenty years. "Fearfully and wonderfully made!"

Day by day and week by week, the developmental process creates a new organ, one cell at a time. Ask yourself, and your doctor, how a FLU shot affects this growth. Could it be possible that as the development of your baby's eye is being engineered, the toxic dump from a flu vaccine could alter the cell development of the eye? Could that lead to a weakness or even a defect? No one can detect this at the time, but it is certainly possible.

Let's consider this a little further. Most chemicals pass through the placenta barrier. Can the placenta differentiate between a street drug and Tylenol? Does the toxic chemical blast from a vaccine seem to stop before entering through the placenta and affecting the unborn child? A mother is told the dangers of alcohol or cocaine but pushed to get a flu shot. This all sounds a little absurd to me – no, VERY absurd!

In a study spearheaded by the Environmental Working Group (EWG) in collaboration with Commonweal, researchers at two major laboratories found an average of two hundred industrial chemicals and pollutants in umbilical cord blood from ten babies born in August and September of 2004 in U.S. hospitals. Tests revealed a total of two hundred eighty-seven chemicals in the group. The umbilical cord blood of these ten children tested harbored pesticides, consumer product ingredients, and wastes from burning coal, gasoline, and garbage.

Among them were eight perfluorochemicals used as stain and oil repellants in fast food packaging, clothes, and textiles including the Teflon chemical PFOA, dozens of widely used brominated flame retardants and their toxic by-products as well as numerous pesticides.
Of the two hundred eighty-seven chemicals detected in umbilical cord blood, we know that:

- One hundred eighty cause cancer in humans or animals.
- Two hundred seventeen are toxic to the brain and nervous system.
- Two hundred eight cause birth defects or abnormal development in animal testing.

Clinical studies tell us that up to 60% of what we put onto our skin makes its way into our bloodstream. Direct absorption through the skin means that substances bypass the body's major filtering organs such as the kidneys and the liver, which would normally assist with toxin removal. Researchers can now demonstrate that once these chemicals enter our own blood stream they can be transferred through to our unborn babies.

This development of life and health begins in the womb and begins with what the mother does to and with her body. Each step along the way is extremely important in the creation of optimal life. For example, when a crack baby is born, the baby is sick and affected by the drugs the mother took as if the baby himself had been on crack. Would we expect a perfect creation from this process? Hardly. The neurological and physical examinations would reveal the problems.

Okay, so we know about crack babies, but what if the mother had been on antidepressant medication and an occasional pain pill? If her child at age five develops vision problems and needs glasses, could we trace it back to the womb where these drugs affected the development of his eyes? What if the child has a physical weakness, immune weakness, or even a behavioral problem? We could possibly trace this all back to the womb and the mother's habits. The moral of the story: We must understand that we need to do our best with a goal of 100% development.

We also know that Mom's stress can affect the unborn child. This means chemical stress, physical stress, emotional stress, and neurological or nerve stress. A chiropractic lifestyle includes reducing and eliminating as many stressors as we can and creating a body full of strength to combat the stress when it is there.

The First Five Years and Beyond

The first year is the most important to set the stage for life, but the immune system needs around seven years to develop into a strong innate healing machine. This development is hindered as the baby is often medicated as early as a day old or within several weeks of birth. A cough, eye mucus, baby rash, or the current craze called acid reflux – and somebody decides to medicate the kid. I've seen infants at two months given Zantac for spitting up when the source can actually be one of two things: one, birth trauma and an interference to the nerve system, primarily the vagus nerve; two, formula which is not close to being like mom's milk (God's natural system for proper development and growth).

Birth trauma is usually the major problem infants face. Most babies are "assisted" in birth by pulling, twisting, or tractioning the head out of the birth canal. In fact, C-section births may require the most forceful pull as the doctor yanks the head to lift the little one out of Mom's tummy. You Tube this and you will see what I mean. Imagine a tiny two-day old baby lying on the floor and a grown man bending over and lifting him up by the head. You'd call the A.C.L.U., CYS, the cops, and anyone else to report this barbaric act of human cruelty, and yet this is what goes on daily in the emergency delivery room.

The birth process is traumatic enough without the pulling and twisting on the delicate baby's head and neck. Did you ever wonder why when we pass an infant to another to hold we instinctively hold the head and neck? Why? We know the importance of head support because we innately know that the spinal cord, or the lifeline, is attached to the head, and if the head flips back without support this could injure the spinal cord, thereby harming the baby. Mom didn't take a course on spinal neurology, yet she innately knows how to handle her baby.

If the spinal vertebra shifts out of its normal alignment, this is called a subluxation. A subluxation will alter proper movement of that area, tense up the muscles attached to the vertebra, and affect the nerve due to tension and inflammation in that area. We have seen many infants unable to turn their head side to side equally due to trauma and subluxation. This can affect the vagus nerve especially, and the vagus nerve goes to all the internal organs, including the tummy!

When someone or some thing irritates the vagus nerve or interferes with its normal neurological output (nerve flow), the tummy or any other organ will not get the correct and full messages from the brain to function. This can lead to acid reflux! So, instead of Zantac with all of its side effects such as headaches, dizziness, constipation, diarrhea, irregular heartbeat, severe stomach pain, or breathing trouble, to name just a few, why not look to the reason WHY this is happening? Have the baby checked immediately for subluxation. Chiropractic care for infants is so gentle and relaxing. Compared to the dangers of medication, it's a no-brainer. Imagine your baby spitting up, getting on Zantac and then dealing with even more severe pain, crying all day and night and suffering from diarrhea and possible heart and breathing problems. These things are LIFE-THREATENING!

In connection with these things, we need to realize that formula food is not optimal food. It is canned vitamins and lots of other unnatural junk, poor substitutions for breast milk. I understand that this stuff is necessary at times, but it's never optimal. People buy their kids the most expensive strollers they can find, dress their infants in designer clothes, and spend a small fortune in decorating their nurseries, but they won't allow these little ones the God-given, free luxury of breast-feeding. It's God's way and therefore the best way, but if you need to use formula, go organic and use the highest quality you can find. This is the vital development of your baby! Go to health stores, consult an expert on infant nutrition, or ask your midwife what is best. Formula food is hard to digest and can often lead to spitting up; so, don't buy into the "acid reflux" diagnosis.

Or do you not know that your body is a temple of the Holy Spirit who is in you, whom you have received from God? You are not your own; you were bought with a price. Therefore honor God with your bodies (1 Corinthians 6: 19-20).

So now we go through the first five years. Antibiotics are given out like candy at times. Antibiotics weaken the immune system and can increase asthma at alarming rates. Your baby needs to develop an immune system on his own. If antibiotics are given, the body's natural ability to build antibodies and proper immune function is altered. Imagine that your baby learns to take his first steps and you see him fall and begin to cry. You say to your spouse, "We need to protect him from falling or feeling bad, so let's put him in a stroller until three or five years old, and then we we'll get him out and let him walk." What would happen? Legs, posture, and all muscular and neurological development would have been stunted, and your child would NEVER be the same. Our children need to develop naturally, have the falls and get back up. That is part of growing up, and it's the same with the immune system. Children need to fight through an infection naturally in order to build their immune system to defend against sickness for life. You can assist by providing proper nutrition, a loving home, a clean environment, and regular visits to the chiropractor to assure a healthy functioning spine and nerve system. As you will learn, each adjustment boosts the immune system and powers the body to heal naturally.

Chiropractic care is not for sickness or to treat a condition. It is to allow your nerve system to function optimally and allow your organs, glands, muscles, structure, and immune system to have full potential. Shouldn't everyone, including our children, have this opportunity?

Their bodies know how to create life in the womb; therefore, shouldn't these same bodies know how to heal from an ear infection or bronchitis? We understand that this amazing system created life inside Mom but tend to forget that this same system can heal on its own when our child has a runny nose and we demand an antibiotic to stop it.

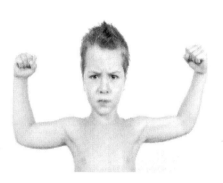

Praise the Lord, O my soul, and forget not all his benefits, who forgives all your sins and heals all your diseases, who redeems your life from the pit and crowns you with love and compassion, who satisfies your desires with good things so that your youth is renewed like the eagle's (Psalm 103:2-5).

This verse says ALL your sins and ALL your diseases. We were made in God's image to be healthy, not sick. We were made in God's image to have the innate strength to fight sickness and diseases. We must honor our body and take care of it naturally.

This allows for optimal development and healing. Not that we may never need medication or a doctor's assistance, but it will be a lot less if we take care of our body naturally in the first place.

Consider the amazing ability the body has to heal itself:

- There are 2.5 trillion red blood cells in your body at any moment. To maintain this number, about two and a half million new ones need to be produced every second by your bone marrow. That's like a new population of the city of Toronto every second.

- Nerve impulses travel up to 200 mph.

- Our heart beats around 100,000 times every day.

- Our blood is on a 60,000-mile journey per day.

- Our eyes can distinguish up to one million color surfaces and take in more information than the largest telescope known to man.

- Our lungs inhale over two million liters of air every day.

- It is believed that the main purpose of eyebrows is to keep sweat out of the eyes.

- A person can expect to breathe in about forty pounds of dust over his lifetime.

This is ALL being done by the brain and nerve system. As we see how intelligent the body is and the accomplishments that are done every second, every minute of every day, how could we possibly think we can duplicate or improve on this by man-made medication or intervention?

Nerve impulses travel from the brain, through the spinal cord, and out the spinal nerve to the connecting body part. For example, the heart beats an average of seventy-two beats per minute, and the brain sends this message to the heart instantaneously throughout the day –every day, every hour and every second. Now if this message would get altered, choked off or interfered with, the heart would not perform properly. The heart may speed up or slow down. When a medical doctor diagnoses this, his normal response is to give a drug to speed up or slow it down. The question ALWAYS is – "Why?" If a subluxation is blocking or interfering with the nerve impulse, this is the very reason for the heart dysfunction. What needs to be done is to restore normal nerve output and get the pressure off the nerve!

I could go on and on about the wonders of our body, from the first five years of life and into old age, and how the medical profession often ignores those wonders. Health does not come from taking medicine, it comes from taking care of your body and allowing it to work the way God designed it. It is interesting that the word "pharmacy" has the word "harm" in it! Look at it this way: Your sickness or lack of health is not a result of lack of chemicals or medications. You don't get a headache because you are void of aspirin. If you suffer from asthma and need to have your lungs refilled before you can breathe, it's not because you have a steroid deficiency, and if you're not sleeping properly it's not because someone neglected to hook you up to a Darth Vader mask or you forgot to take your knockout pills. Whether it's your baby, your teenager, your spouse, or your grandma, a poorly functioning body means that something is lacking in your ABC's.

What a Chiropractic Adjustment Can Do and How It Can Affect Your Life

1. Restore Proper Motion

As I mentioned earlier, the spinal joints can get "locked up" and fixated through trauma, thereby restricting motion. Think of a time when you got out of bed and your neck or back was stiff and you couldn't move it completely. This restriction of motion causes stress to those areas. If your knee didn't have full range of motion, what would happen over time? ARTHRITIS! The same thing happens when your spine gets fixated. Arthritis starts to develop just like when your car is out of alignment and your tires wear out.

Adjustments free up motion and make you feel alive again. This is an amazing part of chiropractic which I have experienced thousands of times. Even in little children, their trauma can restrict motion and cause dysfunction and pain. The adjustment allows for immediate increase in movement and reduction in pain. We experience trauma every day, and it only takes just enough to cause the spine to get "locked up." This can occur with one trauma – baby learning to stand and falling right back on his bum, or daily stressors like sitting in front of the computer and hunching your back, rounding your shoulders, and jutting your head forward for hours. This causes the spine to slowly begin to shift out of alignment, thereby affecting your posture and causing restriction.

Freedom of movement is only one part of an adjustment – but very cool when you experience this for yourself. I remember waking up one day in eighth grade with my neck immobile, stuck to the left. I couldn't even go to school because it hurt so badly; so, I found a neck collar that they gave my mom when she was in a car accident. (By the way, these are horrible because they keep the neck from moving and force it to heal in a crooked position.) I walked around my town, crooked and terribly bored for nearly a week until my neck finally started to move again. Boy, could I have used a chiropractor then!

Adjusting the spine and putting motion in the joint allows for an immediate response of chemicals to be released to relax the muscle and reduce pain. These adjustments have been shown to:

- Increase blood flow
- Increase pain tolerance levels
- Increase range of motion
- Increase the secretion of melatonin and endorphins
- Reduce blood pressure
- Reduce tension and muscle pressure

2. **Reduce Inflammation**

As the joint gets restricted and cannot move freely, inflammation will develop. Inflammation is the normal response to this restriction. The goal is not to reduce inflammation but to restore motion so inflammation goes away naturally. Immediate injury to a joint will cause inflammation to send cox-2 enzymes, which allow for healing and repair, but if the area does not have full range of motion, this can cause a chronic inflammatory state, which leads to breakdown. Anti-inflammatory medications stop the production of cox-2, which restricts the body's natural design to heal!!

Chronic inflammation due to restriction leads to destruction. It's like a slow drip of water on cement. Over time, a big hole will form in the cement floor, just by this little drip; therefore, it is imperative to restore motion and keep all the spinal joints, along with all of your body, moving properly for life.

3. Nerve Output

The spinal nerve, along with the spinal cord, is directly related to motion. A restricted spine becomes inflamed, posture starts to fail, and this can lead to irritation or interference with the nerve output. Think of it this way: Your spinal nerve is like an electrical line in your house with many fibers. If your electrical wire gets frayed or broken, your connection can be affected, and the light or power will be affected. It may flicker or just not work. If this happens, you know that you would have to fix the wiring. What if your fuse box in the basement had one switch off? What would you do if your kitchen lights were out – change the lights, call the electrician, re-wire your kitchen, or start with flipping the switch?

Your spine is your fuse box. If there is pressure on one of the nerves, the connecting body part will not work properly. Nerve output = function. If the nerve is connected to the lungs and there is pressure on that nerve, the lungs cannot function optimally as happened to my wife, Gabrielle. She had asthma from age three to twenty-six, until I went to Life University, discovered this connection, and we decided to give it a try. She had restriction in the area of her neck and back, which supplies the lungs, got adjusted, and in a little over three months she could breathe without medication for the first time in her life. Gabrielle has kept her spine adjusted over the past twenty-four years and continues to be drug-free. Gabrielle's story, along with the stories of countless others, proves that having optimal function of your organs, glands, muscles, and body depends on having an optimally functioning spine and nerve output.

4. Immune Function and Total Health

There is much research about the immune system and chiropractic. Your immune system is controlled by your nerve system; so, it is imperative to have a nerve system free of interference and at high function. Subluxations and a spine not moving and functioning properly will produce stress, and we all know what stress does to the immune system – CRASH!!!

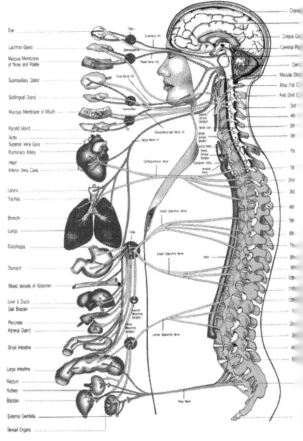

The autonomic nervous system is hardwired into the lymphoid organs such as the spleen, thymus, lymph nodes, and bone marrow that produce the body's immune response. Growing evidence shows that immune function is regulated in part by the sympathetic division of the autonomic nervous system.

In 1975, Ronald Pero, Ph.D., chief of cancer prevention research at New York's Preventive Medicine Institute and professor in Environmental Health at New York University, began researching the most scientifically valid ways to estimate individual susceptibility to various chronic diseases. He has conducted a tremendous amount of research in this area that includes over one hundred sixty published reports in peer reviewed journals. This expertise enabled Pero and his colleagues to discover that various DNA-repairing enzymes could be significantly altered following exposure to carcinogenic chemicals. He found strong evidence that these enzymes could determine an individual's susceptibility to cancer. Lack of those enzymes, Pero said, "definitely limits not only your lifespan but also your ability to resist serious disease consequences."

The relationship between cancer-inducing agents and the endocrine system fascinated Pero. Since the nervous system regulates hormone balance, he hypothesized that the nervous system had to also have a strong influence on one's susceptibility to cancer. To support this argument, he found a substantial amount of literature linking various kinds of spinal cord injuries and cancer. Pero found that these injuries led to a very high rate of lymphomas and lymphatic leukemias. This understanding then led Pero to consider chiropractic care as a means of reducing the risk of immune breakdown and disease.

Pero's team measured one hundred seven individuals who had received long-term chiropractic care. The chiropractic patients were shown to have a 200% greater immune competence than people who had not received chiropractic care and a 400% greater immune competence than people with cancer or serious diseases. Interestingly, Pero found no decline with the various age groups in the study demonstrating that the DNA repairing enzymes were just as present in long-term chiropractic senior groups as they were in the younger groups.

Pero concluded, "Chiropractic may optimize whatever genetic abilities you have so that you can fully resist serious disease...I have never seen a group other than this show a 200% increase over normal patients."

- Spinal lesions, similar to vertebral subluxation complexes caused by misalignments, are associated with exaggerated sympathetic activity, which releases immune regulatory cells into the blood circulation and alters immune function. The nervous system has a direct effect on the immune system due to the nerve supply to the important immune system organs.

- White blood cells, which eat and destroy bad cells, are enhanced through chiropractic care.

- HIV positive patients adjusted over a six-month period showed a 48% increase in CD4 cells, an important immune system component.

- Chiropractic care has been shown to improve serum thiol levels, which measure human health status according to its repair of DNA enzyme activity.

This is amazing research and shows the relationship between a healthy, adjusted spine and immune function. I have seen this happen to many patients through my nineteen years as a chiropractor, and it just amazes me each time. I expect it and still get thrilled by it. Your spine is part of your body that needs to be taken care of. You see now that it is the Master System and needs high priority. You have probably not been taught this during your lifetime. Instead, you were probably taught to wait for sickness, symptoms, or pain to start taking action, and only then did you react to the situation and search for treatment. That is exactly what the pharmaceutical companies and doctors want you to do. This allows them to treat you with their drugs and do massive tests to see WHY you are so sick. The "why" is usually quite simple – you did not take care of your ABC's! So, what is necessary is to reverse your bad habits and restore your health! This is the Chiropractic Principle.

Chiropractic is NOT Stimulation – It's RESTORATION!

The adjustment seems to stimulate healing, and in a way it does because your body will function better, feel better, and perform better after an adjustment; however, it's not about stimulating the nerve, it's about restoring the normal nerve flow to allow healing to occur the way it was designed.

In Stephenson's *Chiropractic Textbook*, he writes: "The chiropractor aims only to restore – to bring about restoration. He adds no more current but removes the obstacles to the normal flow of that which should be supplied to the tissues from the inside. He is able to show how pressure upon nerves can hinder the normal flow and the manner in which he removes the pressure, so that Innate, who is able to attend this body of tissue day and night, may deliver that which is necessary to the organs. The doctor could not give this continuous service, but Innate can. The service of Innate is not stimulation, for stimulation is addition – not restoration."

The ABC's of health is not about adding to or taking away from your body but providing it what it needs to thrive and survive. The medics are all about adding to, taking away, stimulating an organ to work faster or suppressing an organ or blood to work more slowly. It is all about changing the body to look better on tests! The chiropractic approach removes obstacles or interference to allow the body to work properly without drugs to stimulate or suppress.

The Spine and Its Design – Really COOL!

- Protection of the spinal cord: The spinal cord and brain comprise the only system in the body completely surrounded by bone.

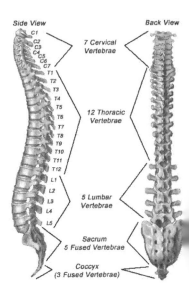

- The spine keeps us upright, and all posture muscles are connected to the spine.

- Your life and energy travel through your spinal cord, supplying healing and function to ALL your body parts and organs.

- Your cerebral spinal fluid travels up and down your spinal cord, which nourishes your brain for growth, and repair, which equals life. The movement in your spine pumps this fluid up and down. That is why proper movement without restriction is critical for brain function. Adjustments keep that fluid moving.

- Your spinal cord is a two-way street. It communicates to the organs to work properly, like giving your stomach the right acid to digest food. Your stomach must first send these messages to the brain to let it know it needs acid production when food hits the stomach – cool two-way communication.

The Science Behind Rebooting Your Brain

Groundbreaking research by Dr. Haavik-Taylor in New Zealand has shown for the first time that the brain and nervous system were stimulated by a chiropractic spinal adjustment. "The process of a spinal adjustment is like rebooting a computer. The signals these adjustments send to the brain, via the nervous system, reset muscle behavior patterns," said Dr. Haavik-Taylor. "By stimulating the nervous system we can improve the function of the whole body. This is something that chiropractors and their patients have known for years, and now we have some scientific evidence to prove it."

Haavik-Taylor was able to measure how brain waves are altered before and after spinal adjustments. This is the first time that anyone has used EEGs to prove that there are definite changes to the way the brain processes information after chiropractic care. This cool two-way communication from spine to brain is why proper spinal movement and alignment are critical for optimal health for both the organs and the brain. By adjusting the spine, we free up interference and thus unblock this communication or nerve flow, thus stimulating or restoring proper nerve output.

Imagine leaving this block there for life – depleting proper nerve output and your highest level of healing. You wouldn't notice it unless it hits a pain nerve, but your body would slowly get weaker or sicker over time. We call it "aging." Don't let it happen to you, and don't accept this terrible myth called "aging."

It is stated that less than 10% of your entire nervous system supplies pain; so, where do the other 90+% of the nerves go? To your muscles, organs, glands, and cells. You could have a severe

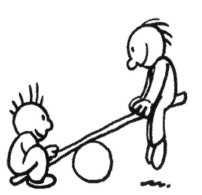

blockage of nerve output and not even know it. This is identified as aging, sickness, low energy or any other dysfunction in your body. Having your spine adjusted and taken care of is a lifelong process. I always say, you can work on your health, or you can work on your sickness.

Sickness care takes a lot more time and money than health care, but we all need to work on our health NOW and not wait for crisis or sickness before we react!

You can't have both sickness and health in your body.
Think of your body's health system as a **seesaw**. One side is sickness, and one side is health. In our office, we work on getting your body so healthy that as your health goes up, your sickness goes down. It always works that way. We don't have to focus on the ten or twenty medications you are on, and how would we even begin to understand that chemical blitz to your body? Instead, we focus on health. Adding health to your body by the ABC's will strengthen and heal your body from the inside out. As your body repairs and heals, less medication is necessary. Trying to get healthy and reversing your habits while continuing to take all the medication is like throwing mud and rocks on your car while someone is washing it.

Lifelong Health

So, how long do you want to be healthy? How long do you have to work on your health? Get adjusted? Eat healthy? Exercise? Have a positive mental attitude? As long as you want to achieve optimal health and healing! The question is sometimes asked, "Do you always have to go to a chiropractor?" Or I've heard people say, "Once you go, you always have to go".

Think of that for just a moment. Do adjustments make you unstable and loosen your spine like a nut and bolt? If so, long-term chiropractic patients and chiropractors would all be like jellyfish. Do we put a hex on you that keeps you coming back, or is it that once you realize how good you feel and how important it is to maintain a healthy spine, you simply want to stay corrected for life?

Let me ask you a bigger question. Does your doctor, who threatens you with your life and demands that you begin taking medicine (poison to your body), tell you that it is only short-term and the medicine will heal you, or does he tell you that you will be on it for life and checked periodically for other problems and given even more drugs, many times for the side effects (newly developed diseases) from the drugs you took in the first place? You know the answer to that question; so, don't ask if you need to be adjusted for life. Instead, ask this question: "What is important for me to do in order to allow my body the most optimal potential for health and healing, and what part do drugs play in this?"

Chiropractic care is similar to church, exercise, eating healthy or drinking H2O – you don't go to church to get something that day – you go to church to honor God and be spiritually healthy throughout your life. *Do not be conformed to this world, but be transformed by the renewal of your mind, that by testing you may discern what is the will of God, what is good and acceptable and perfect (Romans 12:2).*

Finally, brothers, whatever is true, whatever is honorable, whatever is just, whatever is pure, whatever is lovely, whatever is commendable, if there is any excellence, if there is anything worthy of praise, think about these things (Philippians 4:8).

So we do not lose heart. Though our outer self is wasting away, our inner self is being renewed day by day (2 Corinthians 4:16).

How is your inner self, your cells/organs/glands or mind, being renewed each day? Everyday, we must work on our health – spiritually, physically, and mentally. You can be renewed and restored, but it takes a daily commitment to your health – naturally. It will NOT come from medication. The pharmaceutical industry is a business, not a health restoration program, and get this – the medical/pharmaceutical community on research is NOT on short-term care!

A recent article in *Pittsburgh Business Times* in May 2013: "Pitt Researchers Battle With Super Bugs":

- According to the **Food and Drug Administration,** more than seventy percent of the bacteria that cause hospital-associated infections are resistant to at least one type of antibiotic commonly used in treatment.

- About 2 million Americans develop hospital-acquired infections each year, of which nearly 100,000 people die, according to the Infectious Diseases Society of America.

- Drug-resistant infections are a growing problem, and research to develop new antibiotics has been in steady decline since the 1980s, when big pharmaceutical companies started cutting research in that area.

- Because antibiotics are administered for short periods of time, they have become **less lucrative** for pharmaceutical companies that can **make more money on drugs to treat chronic diseases.**

Right from the horse's mouth! Instead of treating the underlying cause, let's develop a vaccine! I understand this logic when the path is money. They are a business, and money is key. In my book, this is not only WRONG but amazingly STUPID. In the immortal words of Forrest Gump: "Stupid is as stupid does."

I take the following verses very strongly when implementing teaching and coaching in my office, at home, and at church:

Not many of you should presume to be teachers, my brothers, because you know that we who teach will be judged more strictly (James 3:1).

So then every one of us shall give account of himself to God (Romans 14:12).

We will be held accountable for what we do and teach, and that's why I teach and practice the following principles for lifelong health:

1. Chiropractic care keeps you healthy. Period.

2. Chiropractic care and the care of our spine needs to be working properly for life, thus allowing optimal healing.

3. The spine and nerve system have the ability to heal your diseases and run your body perfectly. This system is Primary over every other system.

4. Medicine and surgery need to be last on the list.

YOU Decide

Let's take one last look at this amazing body and the role of the nerve system, and you determine just how important it is to you and your family – especially your children. How important is it to move and function optimally? How important is it to use medication sparingly and allow your innate potential to heal and run your body perfectly for life? This next story will show the depths of just how amazing our body is.

In January 2013, my wife, Gabrielle, and I were coming home from town on a cold snowy night. The roads were icy. We were being cautious but able to travel at a decent speed. As we approached a straightaway, I noticed a truck wedged in the rut on the right side of the road. Instantly, I had a bad feeling. Innate identified a problem. The truck bounced out of the rut and shot at my Ford F-150 like a rocket. With no time to maneuver away, we took the hit against my driver's side door. The sound of metal pounding against my truck and tearing away at my side panel was eerie. The power of the truck made us go into a spin. During this spin, Gabrielle screamed out of fear something like, "Oh my God, please help us," and still spinning, I responded back, "We will be okay. Settle down and get hold of yourself."

We spun around one and a half times and lodged into the snowy bank on my side of the road. We were traumatized, to say the least. Gabrielle had been in a leg cast from a broken ankle and a boot for the other severely sprained ankle, so she was extra concerned and horribly afraid that more damage would come to her body. I, on the other hand, felt I had to get control of the situation, the way men do, and somehow make it okay. How I had time to respond is way beyond me! But, let's look behind the scenes at what went on inside our bodies.

When my Innate "felt" something about to happen, my brain immediately went into action. When the truck reached my visual cortex, a trained reflex response directed my foot onto the brake pedal. After that, my hypothalamus ordered up chemicals to launch with lightning speed a series of reactions designed to put me in prime condition to cope with the alarm. Few parts of my body went untouched by the crisis.

First, my vision intensified as my pupils dilated. All my muscles went on alert. Stress hormones affected my entire circulatory system. My heart beat faster, contracting more forcefully, and even in the extremities, vascular muscles relaxed in order to allow blood vessels to widen and carry a greater blood flow. Blood components themselves changed: more blood sugars surged in, providing emergency reserves for working muscles, and clotting materials multiplied in preparation for wound repair. Bronchial tubes flared open to allow faster oxygenation of the blood. In my largest organ, the skin, blood vessels contracted, bringing on a pale complexion ("white as a ghost") but lowering the danger of surface bleeding in case of injury. This reduced volume of circulation in my skin also freed up more blood for the muscles' urgent need. The electrical resistance of skin changed as a protective mechanism against potential bacterial invaders. "Goose-bumps" bulged up all over my body, holding erect millions of hair shafts. Sweat glands poured out assistance to increase the traction of my palms on the steering wheel. Meanwhile, nonessential functions slowed down. Digestion nearly came to a halt – blood assigned to that and to kidney filtration was redeployed for more urgent needs. I wouldn't be able to digest a piece a fruit or try peeing even if I wanted to.

In an external sense, not much damage happened. We were able to get out of the car and assess the damage. The vehicle was totaled; yet, inside my body a full-scale battle was fought and won to equip me for the classic alternatives of "fight or flight." This is a 100% sympathetic response needed for that moment. This trauma to our exterior appeared normal and untouched; however, inside, my spinal alignment was jarred with incredible "whiplash." This shifts the alignment from normal and can lock that area up and put pressure on the delicate nervous system. This subluxation complex that we talked about was now in full swing. Tiny muscles and tendons that connect to my bones and spinal column were microscopically torn apart, creating a release of chemicals to begin healing this area. Inflammation set in and supplied cox-2 enzymes for repair. Pain kicked in, and lack of mobility would soon be apparent. This damage may seem small, but it could've led to severe destruction if not taken care of immediately after a chiropractic assessment.

This classic sympathetic or "flight or fight" response is necessary for battle. This is all initiated and controlled by your brain in a flash of your seventy-five trillion cells to perform perfectly. My first response, by applying my foot to the brake, resulted from a direct command of the nervous system. Long ago, when I first learned to drive, my brain sorted out the sequence of nerve firings required for me to lift my foot and slide it to the left, and to turn the steering wheel with short, jerky motions. During the accident, however, I didn't have to think about this critical response. In a moment of stress, my brain relied on a memory bank of programmed responses and sent high-speed orders along nerve pathways. The orders were very specific to my foot muscles and wrist muscles; however, the other complex reactions – the heart rate, skin changes, respiratory adjustments – occurred because of the hormonal system. My brain initiated an order to a gland, in this case the adrenal, to secrete a chemical messenger into the bloodstream. The hormone does not deliver a message as immediate, precise, and definite as the nerves, but in a few seconds it was able to reach every cell in my body. Fear, relief, heightened awareness – I felt all these sensations, and for the next few hours my body was much more alert and responsive to my environment.

As we think about what happened in just a split second, it is overwhelmingly amazing. My Innate, God-supplied reactions were all orchestrated beautifully inside. I didn't have to think or coordinate this hormonal or neurological response. It just worked. We are designed that way. It is all programmed in your nervous system. If this system is allowed to work without interference (subluxation – the trauma Gabrielle and I had during this event), then our bodies can coordinate healing all day, every day.

The same is true for everyday events. We get bad news and our heart starts to pound and hands start to sweat. We need to catch ourselves from falling when we trip over a bump in the rug. Our heart needs to speed up and lungs need to pump more oxygen in times of stress to supply healing and repair before damage sets in. These and millions of internal responses are happening every second in your body. Your immune organs and glands killing invaders before an infection overtakes your lungs is just one primary example of how your body heals without your even knowing it.

This is the true essence of vitalistic health and healing. Chiropractic care is not about the 10% nerves that supply pain. It is about a body in full response to the environment because of a nerve system free of interference, which allows for optimal healing. When you accept this as fact and truth, you will appreciate the role of your nerve system as truly the Master System, thus creating a heightened sense of the importance to take care of this system from birth until the day you meet your Maker. And yet you may ask, "Does my insurance pay for this?" How foolish this sounds when we understand the magnitude and importance of this incredible nervous system! You are the gatekeeper of your temple, not the insurance company and certainly not a doctor. A doctor follows advice from his medical school knowledge and what the drug companies tell him. Remember, the doc went to MEDICINE school. He does NOT consult the God-given, innate knowledge from your body.

Beware of the scribes, who like to walk around in long robes, and love greetings in the marketplaces and the best seats in the synagogues and the places of honor at feasts, who devour widows' houses and for a pretense make long prayers. They will receive the greater condemnation (Luke 20:46-47).

That verse speaking of how the Pharisees acted in public reminds me of how the pharmaceutical companies and all their marketing strategies behave. They stick out their chest and pound them with great vigor over the wonders of medicine but yet neglect the innate potential for the body to heal without all their moneymaking chemicals.

Then they asked Him, "Where is your father?" "You do not know Me or My Father," Jesus replied. "If you knew Me, you would know My Father also" (John 8:19).

I often imagine the Pharisees standing around Jesus and not having a clue who He really is. I can't but compare it to our modern day health care system (which is really nothing but sick care) and how it has affected us. We stand in the presence of our amazing self-healing body, and we don't even take the time to respect it but immediately inject it with vaccines and antibiotics the minute we are born and continue to do this throughout our lives because the "doctor" tells us to. People, it's about time we respect our body and respect our Innate Intelligence. This would be the biggest turning point in our health history if we allowed this. How will this begin to happen? It first starts with you and your family. It starts with me and my house, my office, and my patients. That is why I write. That is why I am on a mission to get this message out. That is what God programmed me to do and to be.

As I read Isaiah 61:1-2, I apply this to my mission and what has called me to do: *The spirit of the Sovereign Lord is on me, because the Lord has anointed me to proclaim good news to the poor. He has sent me to bind up the brokenhearted, to proclaim freedom for the captives and release from darkness for the prisoners. To proclaim the year of the Lord's favor.*

We all have a purpose, and that's mine. I feel blessed to understand these principles because they have saved my life and the future health of my family, and I live to impart these things to you. This is your year of God's favor. This is the time to turn in a new direction and be blessed with amazing health. This is the year that medication ceases and your body returns to good health.

Mechanistic vs Vitalistic

It comes down to Choice. Two paths.

Mechanistic is mechanical type thinking. Blood pressure high – take a chemical to lower it. Sugar levels too high – take insulin to lower it. Short term fixes compared to correcting the underlying problem. This belief is really devaluing or underestimating the power to heal; the power of your body restoring itself without the use of drugs or surgery. That each individual part or organ of your body is independent of all others and needs to be addressed. Pain relief for the moment. Addressing a symptom rather than the correction.

Vitalistic belief is that your body, and all living systems, are self-regulating, self-repairing, and self-healing. God designed the universe to run itself without our help. The sun comes up, the sun goes down. Flowers grow as the rain supplies the water, the sun supplies the energy and the soil supply the environment. We don't have to help the universe work better, nor could we. We need to get out of the way and stop interfering. This is also true for your body.

Vitalism understands that the power that made the body is the power that heals the body. This power is creating at conception and directs our steps until the moment we pass into God's arms. This Innate power and wisdom knows exactly how to control our blood pressure, heal a cut, drive sugar out of our blood stream, or create energy from the apple you ate at lunch. It does not need help; it needs us to stop interfering and get out of the way.

Your body is at constant work to supply balance and health to your body. It knows how to do this at magnificent precision. We as humans, and as doctors, will never truly understand how powerful and perfect our bodies are. As a Vitalistic Chiropractor, I believe your body has amazing talent to heal itself and restore health no matter where you may be in your health journey. But it is up to you to restore and not suppress symptoms. The ABC's restore. Medicine simply covers up your body trying to tell you that you have a problem.

Medical Treatment	Chiropractic Care
Blood based	Nerve based
Treats symptoms	Corrects cause
Renders sickness care	Offers health care
Prescribes drugs	Makes adjustments
Sees body as parts	Sees whole person
Removes organs	Revives organs
Kills germs	Helps resist germs
Causes side effects	Produces positive effects
Artificial	Natural
Risky	Safe

Chiropractic care as you have read, goes well beyond the stiff neck or sore back problem. It addresses life and health as a whole. We know that God made your body and God heals your body, and we do all we can to restore your body to the original design and let this power heal and restore.

Believe and implement your ABC's! Your life is precious, given by God. Allow it to function the way HE designed. That is the Chiropractic Principle and the Chiropractic Lifestyle. This is your road to health.

TESTIMONIES:

REAL LIFE, REAL PEOPLE

In the mouth of two or three witnesses shall every word be established (2 Corinthians 13:1).

God only requires two or three witnesses to confirm the truth and validity of something. Maybe you require more. If so, I have a lot of witnesses who will verify for you that the things I've been telling you in this book are absolutely true.

Perhaps you've talked with people who have told you that they tried these things I'm talking about and that these things don't work, but I can pretty much promise you that they're not telling you the whole story. Remember the four-legged chair? You need ALL of the legs, and I'm quite certain that the naysayers aren't using all of them. For example, Uncle Joe decides to change his **attitude** and believe only the best about his health. He talks like Norman Vince Peale (positive speaking) and goes to church several times a week to claim his healing. These aren't necessarily bad things, but these things alone aren't going to cut it, and Uncle Joe is not your best witness. Don't enter his testimony into the court record.

Then there's your co-worker, Susie, who decides to change her **behavior**. She buys a slew of nutritional books and spends a small fortune in health food stores. She joins the gym, dragging herself out of bed at 7:00AM every morning so she can work her abs, glutes, pecs, delts, etc. Not bad stuff, but, again, not all four legs of the chair. Susie is not your star witness.

Then you have your neighbor, Fred, who goes to a **chiropractor** for a period of time, or maybe just periodically, and continues to suffer in the long run as he complains about his health, is a couch potato, and lives on Big Macs and Fritos. He tells you what quacks all chiropractors are and how much money he threw down the drain. I obviously believe in chiropractic, but you don't want to sit on the chair if that's its only leg. Fred is on a shaky foundation and doesn't deserve to be on the stand.

Uncle Joe, Susie, and Fred – if those are the kinds of witnesses you've been listening to, you need to consider that they're probably not telling you the whole story. There are missing pieces to these weak testimonies, and you need to throw these witnesses out of your courtroom.

So now, let's bring in some credible witnesses – real life, real people who have practiced the ABC's of health and are sitting on a solid foundation. Hear their testimonies, slam your gavel, and render your verdict.

Mother Knows Best

I met Dr. Tressler in 1994, when we both worked in the same chiropractic office. Dr. Tressler left to open his own practice as I stayed on at the previous practice. Our paths had crossed many times over the years, but in 2005, he asked me if I would be interested in working for him at his office. As I was working in the medical field at that time and was tired of seeing those patients suffering with conditions that I knew chiropractic care would benefit, I decided to accept his offer and return to the profession I have come to love.

My love affair with chiropractic started when I answered an ad for a part-time chiropractic assistant's job in 1993. Next to getting married to my husband, Tim, and having my children, Ashley, 24, and Cody, 21, this was the best decision of my life. I thank GOD every day that He led me to the chiropractic lifestyle and specifically to Dr. Tressler.

As a young mother, I remember having an uneasy feeling about vaccines and "routine" medical trips to the pediatrician's office for "well" visits, asking myself, "Why, if my children are healthy, would they need to go to an office full of sick kids just to be told that they were healthy when I already knew they were?"

Tim and I decided to stop the madness, and we quit taking our kids in for these useless visits, which meant no more vaccines either. As a result, we were asked to leave the practice, and the reasoning was that we were not following their "guidelines" and were putting other children at the office at risk because our kids weren't vaccinated. At the time, it didn't make sense, but I now know the full reasoning behind their statements. That, however, is another topic that would take forever to go over. IF you ever want to talk about that, stop at the office, and I will be more than happy to enlighten you on their "guidelines."

At about the same time that we left that pediatric practice, I answered the ad about the part-time chiropractic position and got the job which began in November of 1993. In the spring of 1994, I went to my first of many chiropractic seminars, and it transformed my life. Dr. Sigafoose was the first person I ever heard speak about the true chiropractic message, and I changed my life right then and there. I have never looked back. He explained to me how the body uses fevers to heal itself and that inside every single living person is a healing ability that is unmatched in any medical field. This healing ability is named INNATE. I was sold!!! It was exactly what I always knew but never really understood until Dr Sigafoose explained it to me so beautifully and with such simplicity. This is why, as that young mother, I always had that uneasy feeling about vaccines and such. It was my "innate," God speaking to me, telling me that there is a better way.

My family's life has never been the same. We are happy, healthy, and live the chiropractic lifestyle. It has not always been easy to stay on the path, but I have persevered through many challenges, whether they are simple or more complicated. I have and I will always stay true to what Dr. Sigafoose taught me: YOUR BODY IS SELF-HEALING AND THE POWER THAT MADE THE BODY HEALS THE BODY.

My children have only ever been rarely sick, and if they did get something, they got over it more quickly and naturally without medical interference. This was not because they were "lucky." It was because I put hard work into choosing to follow the chiropractic lifestyle that had been taught to me all those years earlier.

Never had this lifestyle been put to the test more than with my father. In 2003, my father was diagnosed with emphysema, which is now called COPD. He was told he had to get on at least three medications immediately for treatment and to come back within three months for more testing to see if they needed to add any more medications. This was unacceptable to me, as it went against everything that I have learned over the past ten years. We were going to go down a different path. My family had very strong feelings about my choosing to not let my dad be on meds, but as they weren't the ones taking him to all the doctor appointments, let's just say, they had no choice in the matter. I convinced my dad to start getting adjusted more consistently, and because he refused to change his diet, I added in natural supplements and special herbs to help him with his breathing.

We went back to the doctor every six months for eight years for routine testing, and not until the last two years did he need any medication to aid in his breathing. Reluctantly, I agreed to let him take the meds, agreeing that they were needed at that time to help him breathe. The medical doctor was dumbfounded that he was not on multiple meds and not worse each time we would go in for his appointment. They would always recommend the latest greatest new drug for him to try, but I always stood firm on by belief that THE POWER THAT MADE THE BODY HEALS THE BODY. My dad proved that, and each time I would tell the medical doctor that we would not be taking their new drug of choice, he would say, "I guess whatever you're doing is working, as he should probably not be living at this point".

My response would always be, "What do mean – you 'guess'? What I'm doing IS working." Then I would tell him that the biggest thing my dad had added was getting adjusted more frequently, etc. The doctor never really gave the chiropractic principle credit for saving my dad, but I know that was the reason.

Sadly, my dad passed away in September of 2011, not from breathing issues but from cancer that was never picked up on by any of the number of tests he had every six months for eight years. When I called the doctor to tell him that my dad had passed, he said that what I did for my dad gave him eight years of life that he should have never had and noted how my decision not to medicate my dad could have been the reason. At least I got him to admit something.

I am going to speak out about the chiropractic principle until GOD calls me back home again. It is my life's work. It is important that everyone on the planet has the opportunity to hear the message as I did all those years ago. I will never back down from the truth. The chiropractic lifestyle that I learned and adapted for my family and myself will never fail, ever!!! Be strong and stay true to the principle, and you will have the most abundant life possible.

Wendy Doerzbacher, Harrison City Pa

Croup, Chiropractic, and now Cats!

Our son, Cameron, was very allergic to cats and got croup cough constantly. When he ended up in the emergency room because of croup, we knew we needed to do something different to avoid the life of chronic doctor visits and medications. Once he started regular chiropractic care, Cameron no longer got as sick with croup and hasn't been back to the emergency room. We are also fortunate to have two beautiful cats in our home, and he now has no allergy to them. Chiropractic works!

The Swartz Family, Delmont Pa

More Amazing than Houdini

On New Year's Day, 2012, my husband and I decided to sign up for Weight Watchers. We both wanted to lose weight. After two months of doing their plan, neither one of us was having any great success. Very discouraged, John was reading the Plum Advance Leader newspaper one Saturday morning in February and saw Dr. Tressler's ad. John called the office immediately to sign us up for a workshop.

We both came to the workshop to listen, and, after hearing all of the information; we thought it was too good to be true. Both of us wanted to lose weight and also get off the medicines we were taking. John was taking eleven different ones, and I was taking three. I struggled with weight my whole life and tried all kinds of plans, and both of us even got hypnotized a few years back. All of that, including the Houdini stuff, proved useless; so, we both started Dr. Tressler's plan, customized for us. After just a few days, we were seeing great results and felt awesome. John lost 86 pounds and 18% body fat and has reduced his medicine from eleven to one and feels great, outworking guys who are way younger than he is. I lost 116 pounds and 18% body fat and do not take any medicine anymore. In just nine months, I feel great.

The program is truly amazing, and we both regained our health back, thanks to Dr. Tressler and his staff. I now work with Dr. Tressler as a weight loss coach to help others regain their health and reach their weight loss goals. John and I both continue to get regular chiropractic adjustments and live a healthy lifestyle and both feel better than we have in years.

John and Sandy Seman, Plum Boro Pa

My Child was Trapped in a Dying Body

Colton was born on November 19th, 2001, with a hole in his heart and a restricted heart valve. We knew the night he was born that he would have to have open-heart surgery at approximately six months of age to correct those problems. At a little over two months, Colton was scheduled to receive his first set of vaccines. I had heard of the dangers, the risk of heavy metals, possible connections to autism, etc., but also knew that in four to five months he would be admitted to Children's Hospital for his surgery where there would be children who had some of the illnesses that these vaccines were supposed to protect him from. I talked at length with my pediatrician about the risks and specifically questioned the ingredients in the actual bottles of vaccines that would be given to Colton. He assured me that there was no thimerosal (mercury) in the vaccines that they used and that, in his opinion, the risks were greater to admit Colton to the hospital for his surgery without the shots; so, I got him the first set of vaccines on January 28, 2001.

Exactly seventeen days later, problems started when Colton woke up one morning with a red patch of skin on the left side of his face that was all bubbled up and oozing a clear yellowish liquid. My immediate concern was that this liquid was running into his left eye. Of course, it was a Saturday, and the pediatrician's office was closed, so the nurse on call advised me to take him to Children's Hospital. My husband and I, trusting that they knew more than we did, listened to that advice. We sat in the emergency room there for over 6 ½ hours, finally saw a doctor, and after looking at his face for all of thirty seconds, he said he didn't know what it was or what would have caused it but all we had to do to cure it was put 2% hydrocortisone cream on it three times a day for five days. We did that, it cleared up, and then a few days after we stopped using the cream, it came back. This time it was worse, and more and more spots and blotches began breaking out all over his face, shoulders and chest. Again, not knowing what else to do, I took Colton back to the pediatrician. I asked him if this could be a reaction to the vaccines, and he assured me it was not. I then stated my opinion that **something** caused it – he was not born with these spots all over him. I asked if it could be possible that his neck was too straight because of the difficult forceps delivery he had had and if that could potentially be the cause of these problems. He told me he had never heard of that. He diagnosed him with having eczema, told me it was a very common childhood "ailment," and recommended I take him to a dermatologist for specialized treatment.

We saw the dermatologist, and she agreed with the pediatrician that it was only eczema, and the only treatment was steroid cream and antihistamines. She prescribed a 5% steroid cream, which I had to smear on the rash, then put a wet onesie over him and then dress him in dry clothes on top of that to increase the absorption of the steroid into his skin. She also prescribed Zyrtec, an antihistamine, which we gave to him at night to supposedly help him sleep – which, by the way, never worked. I followed that protocol for a month, the eczema went away, but with three or four days of stopping the cream, it came back, and this time it was spreading to his legs and the underside of his arms and armpits. Around this time is when the itching became unbearable for him. He would scratch so hard and so long that he would begin to bleed. This is when we started putting socks – or as we called them, "puppets" – on his hands to prevent the constant scratching.

It was at this point in time that I began investigating chiropractic care. We took Colton to several chiropractors for adjustments, muscle testing, and meridian treatments. They were all adamant about that fact that his condition was due to the vaccines he had received. His condition improved slightly but then reached a plateau.

At seven months old, Colton underwent the open-heart surgery. He came through that with flying colors, and for several weeks after the surgery had no rash whatsoever. We thought it was all behind us, and then a short time later it reared its ugly head again – now worse than ever. Keep in mind that in the five days he was in the hospital, his little body was invaded by thirty-two different medicines. There has to be a connection, right? Common sense says so, but the entire medical profession kept telling us "no way."

When he began eating solid foods, Colton's condition still worsened. His hands, wrists, and arms swelled up and stayed swollen. Every food he ate, except green beans and yellow squash, caused a flare-up in the itchiness and redness. The pediatrician now recommended allergy testing to determine specific foods and/or environmental irritants causing the problem. When I explained the severity of the condition to the allergist, he thought I was "off my rocker." After some heated words, though, he ran all the antibody tests. Lo and behold, the tests showed Colton was "allergic" to corn, potatoes, peas, wheat, milk, eggs, oats, barley, all meat, peanuts, Brussels sprouts, beets, tomatoes, cats, dogs, and – believe it or not – polyester! He would even flare up from odors in stores like J.C.Penney and Wal-Mart.

For almost a year and half, Colton literally survived on a diet consisting exclusively of green beans, yellow squash, mushrooms, a few lentil beans, and rice milk! As time went on, he broke out even more on his stomach, his neck, and even inside his little ears. He was wearing his puppets now almost twenty-four hours a day, every day.

We bought a new sweeper specifically made to remove the smallest micrograms of allergens the home. We also bought a special air cleaner, installed a reverse osmosis system on our water faucet, put our cats outside, cleaned all the carpets, had all the walls washed, changed soaps and laundry detergent, and literally washed every piece of clothing and bedding in the house in the new "chemical free" formula. Nothing helped!

We then heard of another doctor who practiced alternative medicine and began taking Colton there twice a week (a two-hour round trip drive). Through computer testing and Bioset frequency treatments, his office was the next to tell us that Colton was indeed suffering from vaccine damage and heavy metal poisoning. The toxins in the vaccines had literally eaten holes through his intestinal wall, and his immune system was completely wiped out. The diagnoses given were "leaky gut syndrome" and a severe yeast infection. Because there were actual holes in his intestinal wall, when Colton would eat food, it would leak out of his intestines into his body. His body viewed it as a foreign object and therefore tried to "fight it off" so to speak, thereby causing the reaction of redness, itching, and sometimes hives. We began giving him supplements to detox the metals, help him digest fats, and heal his intestinal tract. We saw progress, but after a while, he plateaued again. The one condition we were unable to cure was the yeast infection. The doctor prescribed Diflucan, which we gave to Colton for about a month, but even that didn't kill the yeast.

Finally, by the grace of God, in September of 2003, we found Dr. Tressler's office! We learned that the reason Colton had such a high level of yeast is because the body produces yeast to fight off mercury poisoning. The yeast bonds to the mercury to prevent it from getting into the brain! We realized at that point that God was actually protecting Colton from poisoning to his brain by preventing the yeast from being killed! I was still, however, extremely skeptical, as I had already tried several other chiropractors. But, knowing that giving up on my child was absolutely NOT an option, I took Colton in for x-rays at Dr. Tressler's, and wouldn't you know, Colton's neck was perfectly straight, and he also had a slight curve in his spine! We immediately began treatment on Colton, and the rest of our family, and we all saw immediate improvement. There were periods of time, sometimes only five or ten minutes, but times nonetheless, where you could see the redness calm down or notice him not trying to scratch as much. We changed his milk from rice milk to raw goat's milk, put him on a number of natural supplements, including 4:1 oil, primrose oil, and trace minerals. We did Asyra testing and used homeopathic drops. Gradually,

Colton's periods of relief started increasing to twenty to thirty minutes, and every once in a while we'd get a whole day of no scratching. It was a true miracle! In three months, Colton's neck curve was perfect, and it was obvious to everyone that he was feeling much better.

We had also taken Colton to see Dr. Patricia Kane in Philadelphia to see if she could shed any more light on Colton's case, as she was a so-called "expert" in the area of detoxification. She ran a battery of tests, as well as blood work, and on December 23rd of 2003, her office called to tell us the bad news that Colton's blood work did not look very good. She saw indications of potential bone tumors and possible kidney failure looming. Needless to say, I was an instant basket case. Dr. Kane's office referred us to Dr. Cartaxo, a pediatric specialist in New Jersey. We drove to New Jersey and met with Dr. Cartaxo who was much more concerned about the fact that Colton was missing out on tactile development because of having to wear the socks on his hands. It concerned her more than the blood work. Her solution for helping him was to put him on internal hydrocortisone. Frustrated once again with no answers, we came home and vowed to do no more blood work, no more cortisone – only chiropractic! The only doctor's office that never quit or gave up on Colton's hope of becoming well was Dr. Tressler's office!

Colton is now completely cured! We had been living with a baby boy who was never happy when he woke up in the morning like most babies are. He woke up crying every day and saying, "I itchy, Mommy...I itchy!" He never slept more than two to three hours per night, physically lying on top of me so I could hold his hands apart to keep him from scratching, because he was soooo itchy. Those two to three hours of sleep were broken up by fifteen minutes of sleep, then up for an hour or so, then fifteen minutes more sleep, then up again, and on and on and on. The summer of 2003 was agonizing. On those hot summer days; Colton wore long pants, long-sleeved shirts, socks on his hands that reached to the top of his arms, and sometimes turtlenecks just to keep him from scratching and bleeding. He couldn't even stand to put his little feet in a swimming pool because the water burned him so badly.

Today, Colton is a different child. He is a healthy, vibrant seven-year-old who sleeps all night and wakes up with a big smile on his face, wanting to go outside and throw water balloons. He loves school, playing with his dog, and jumping on his trampoline. He's able to wear not just short-sleeved shirts, but tank tops, NO puppets ever, and shorts and sandals! He loves to swim in pools and the ocean! And... he actually sleeps all night without socks on his feet. These things, which to most people are no big deal, are true miracles to us, even years after the fact!!!

Colton's heavy metal poisoning and his depleted immune system and digestive system obviously led to severe nutritional deficiencies. On top of that, he had the structural problems with his neck and spine. Once the structural repair chiropractic treatments began, the metals began to disappear, and his immune system and digestive system were built up, and his food "allergies" began disappearing as well. Today, he can eat everything except nuts and peas. Another miracle!

Contrary to the Elidel commercial you hear on television, there **is** a cure for eczema – it's called structural repair chiropractic care and proper nutrition! I believe these two things in combination with each other can cure any ailment out there – IF people are willing to do whatever it takes to achieve the result. You can't let ANYTHING stop you – not money, not time, not lost sleep, not even tears – nothing! There **is** an answer, and things can get better, but you cannot quit! God does not permit bad things to happen without good coming from them, and believe it or not, we have seen much good. Our faith has grown, our eating habits have improved, our entire view of health-care has changed, and our priorities have been realigned.

All that matters in the big scheme of things is that Colton now has a bright, healthy life ahead of him. Always keep the end result in mind, and don't **ever** give up on finding <u>your</u> cure.

Doctor Tressler has been Heaven sent to all of us. He is an angel here on this earth, and if you trust him and follow his guidance, God will work miracles through him for you, too, just as he did for us!

Lu Ann Ryniec, Oakmont Pa

His Mission IS Possible

We started coming to Dr. Tressler's office about 2 months and 45 pounds ago. Before we came we had an interest in and an appreciation for chiropractic, but when we heard Dr. Tressler and his staff talk about it we finally began to understand it. Chiropractic is fundamentally about design; specifically that God designed our body-mind-heart-spirit to be healthy.

When we make life choices that are contrary to the design we become broken-disjointed-disconnected. When God promises to bless His people, to redeem and reconcile and restore them, that's not just spiritual its psychological and physical as well. God wants to restore the years the locusts have eaten, to redeem the time lost to foolish decisions. This is the mission of Dr. Tressler and his staff; to see people restored to the health God always intended them to have by embracing the beautiful simplicity of design. Its has been a pleasure and an honor to have my family be their patients.

- Rev Dr Joshua C. Strunk, MDiv., EdD.

One Last Try Changed My Life

I have tried many ways to lose weight over the past recent years. Since it was so difficult to lose, I figured that at my age there wasn't much else I could do. Hormones must be ruling my body. Then I heard about a homeopath. I thought, might as well go see what he could do for me. I would try one more thing to lose weight. I bought lots of vitamins, and he told me to eat better. That's it. I lost no weight.

I heard a radio personality recommend a diet shake and thought, might as well try it. After four weeks of eating one meal a day, I lost a whopping three pounds. That's it. I gained it back and then some.

Then I heard a Bizburgh radio segment on my way home from work. It sounded too good to be true, but I thought, might as well call. What could it hurt to try one last time?

Skeptical, I entered their office. The staff, which I had never met before, greeted me with smiles, making me feel welcome. I was scanned and x-rayed and given a consultation. They recommended a total wellness plan for me to follow. Hey, wait a minute. I had only come in for weight loss help, but now they suggested a total plan. What they were telling me made sense, though. There was so much information to absorb, but I thought, might as well go all out this one last time.

Now, after going through a forty-day weight loss, detox plan and regularly visiting the office for adjustments, and actually doing the home rehab, I can say without a doubt that this was and still is the best choice I could have made. Dr. Tressler and Dr. Barto and all of the staff have been nothing less than supportive and encouraging to me every step of the way. They help me understand my body, and at no time do I feel my questions are stupid or annoying. I am now one of the smiling faces when I visit their office, but, more than that, I am smiling inside, also. I crave exercise. I can walk through the grocery store and wonder how I put all that junk food and chemicals in my body without thought.

I am fifty-one years old and feel better than I have in a long time. Yes, I lost those stubborn twenty pounds I carried for years, but more important than that is what I have gained. I have respect for my body. I have confidence in myself. I have the knowledge to make wise choices. I have a support team willing to ensure my success. Sure, I will treat myself to all the abundance life has to offer, but I know what I need to do and I am confident I will not gain that weight back. I will continue to strengthen my muscles and strive to be the best I can be. You know, you only live once; so, might as well live it to the fullest.

Anita Hagey, Lower Burrell Pa

91 Lbs. Gone in 6 ½ months

I just wanted to say that this was one of the best decisions I made in my whole life. I have been on so many diets over the years, but Dr. Tressler's program is not just a diet. It's an overall health changer. I have never felt this good, even since my twenties. I have lost 91 Lbs. in just 6 ½ short months.

I was in a car accident and was going from doctor to doctor because of all the pain I was in. After only a few weeks of seeing Dr. Tressler, my health started improving more and more. With both chiropractic care and a real weight loss and health plan; today, I feel better than ever.

Thank you Dr. Tressler, Dr. Barto, and staff for helping me.

Shirley Graham, New Stanton Pa

Insomnia Defeated

For two years, I suffered from insomnia. I would either go to bed and toss and turn for hours, or I would go right to sleep for thirty to forty-five minutes, then be up for most of the night. My doctor had me try Sleepy-Time Tea, melatonin and valerian root. Nothing worked! He finally prescribed Ambien CR, which worked but was expensive, and I worried about becoming addicted to a prescription sleep-aid.

The night after my first adjustment, I slept well, but I wasn't ready to believe it was because of being adjusted. After sleeping well for a week, I told Dr.Tressler that he must have been doing something right! It has been two months now, and I have had no sleeping problems since coming to Dr.Tressler.

Alice, Madison Pa

From Narcotics to Singing Birds

As a nurse in training thirty years ago, it was never stated outright; however, we were taught that medical treatment should always supersede chiropractic treatment. Chiropractic treatment involved short-term adjustments and "bone crushing." I was reluctant to fall for the "new wave" of chiropractic treatment. Today, I believe it should go hand in hand with medical treatment. Rule out serious disease with your M.D., but you owe it to yourself to listen to Dr. Tressler's theories firmly based in education which describes the body's own healing methods. I wish I had begun years ago.

Eighteen years ago, as a young mother of two boys, I was diagnosed with fibromyalgia, a chronic muscular pain condition that occurs throughout the body. It is believed to have begun with the Epstein Barr Virus as a result of untreated strep. I had chronic muscle spasms in my shoulders and pain in my cervical spine. My shoulders were as hard as a wood surface, and it affected my daily life. Muscle relaxants are typically prescribed but can't be taken during the day. Chronic Fatigue Syndrome soon followed.

Chronic Fatigue Syndrome is strange. You are tired until it is time to sleep and then become insomniac. The prescription is sleeping pills. It is an endless cycle, sleeplessness = pain. My blood pressure spiked to 210/100, and I began to take two blood pressure medications. In addition, I take a cholesterol-lowering drug and have been diagnosed with Type II Diabetes, which I have been able to control by diet. People who have experienced it have told me that, with proper and ongoing chiropractic treatment, many of these medications will be reduced or even eliminated.

During this period of time, I have bounced between gynecologists, internists, endocrinologists, rheumatologists, seven chiropractors, four physical therapists, and my fabulous family physician who is thrilled at my newfound energy levels. Other chiropractors took no x-rays, spent no time educating me, did not outline a course of therapy and, like the physical therapists, offered relief for thirty minutes. Six months ago, my medications included thyroid medication, muscle relaxants, prescription strength NSAID's (Ibuporphan, Ultram, Aleeve, etc. type medications), calcium and potassium for muscle spasms, cholesterol lowering and high blood pressure medications, and, of course, sleeping medications and occasionally anti-anxiety medication to help me relax enough to go to sleep. Most recently, narcotics were prescribed to help alleviate the pain. As a result of the medications, it is necessary for me to get expensive and extensive blood work quarterly to monitor the effect of the medication in my liver and other vital organs.

As a fifty-five year old looking forward to the "empty nest" and a positive senior life, I found that when a friend or family member suggested an evening outing, I required a nap during the day and

103

hoped for the best. Generally, after a two-mile walk in the park, my muscles were in agony for two days.

I came upon an ad for Tressler Chiropractic one day: "DR. I CAN'T GO ON LIKE THIS." .

Dr. Tressler and his staff explained that if it took eighteen years to get in this condition, it would take some time to return my body to the way it was meant to be. This outstanding team of well-educated staffers explains daily what is required for proper treatment in order for my body to heal itself. My treatment plan was for sixteen weeks of intense therapy to return my spine to its original position, as evidenced by x-rays, followed up by in-office therapy, as well as exercises to complete at home. Within two weeks, I experienced a 25% improvement in my spinal curvature. Once my cervical spine is in proper alignment, I will begin maintenance adjustments for life. My goal is to live with this condition and reduce my medications. I need to do my part and follow the exercise regiment for life. I also hope to work again, which I gave up two years ago.

After a few weeks, I began to wake with the birds! I hadn't awakened before 10 AM in years. I lost weight, without trying. Then came the first amazing day when I awoke, and for the first time in years, FELT NO PAIN. It doesn't happen every day, but I feel like I have hope for the rest of my life. My pain medication is reduced by 50%. I go to my M.D. for blood work soon, and I am anxious to see the results. My only regret is that I didn't begin to see Dr. Tressler earlier.

Have I told you how long I have been in treatment with Dr. Tressler? Six weeks. I now look forward to the rest of my life. I am thrilled when I see young children getting adjusted. As Dr. Tressler tells me...my results are only "the tip of the iceberg." I CAN'T WAIT!

Jane, Murrysville Pa

Thank God for the Traffic Light

I am sixty-five years old. I have had arthritis issues for many years. I have had two knee and two hip replacements because of severe degeneration of my joints. After my last knee replacement, I was convinced that my problems were solved; however, I then experienced a terrible, chronic pain in my lower back. The left side of my body was so weak that I had to walk with a cane. I was unable to be on my feet for more than fifteen minutes without finding a chair and sitting down. I couldn't shop in stores that didn't have carts that I could use for support. I had to walk up and down stairs holding on to railings for dear life and taking them one foot at a time. I visited an orthopedist and a rheumatologist. Their solution to the problem was to put me on more drugs.

One day this past August, as I was sitting at the traffic light beside the Tressler Chiropractic office, something on his sign drew me in for an evaluation. Now, six months later, I am free of the terrible back pain and am able to climb stairs in a normal fashion. In addition, I have made some nutritional adjustments, which are helping me to have more energy and lose weight. Finally, through the help of a personal trainer, I am exercising at least three days a week and have developed considerable strength, but one of the things I am really thrilled about is that when I am driving and have to change lanes in traffic, I can actually turn my head enough that I can do so easily and safely. (I used to have to shift my entire body so that I could see out of the back of the car, and I've had many really close calls as a result).

I am grateful to God for nudging me into making the stop at Tressler Chiropractic, and I am grateful to Dr. Tressler and his staff for their help and expertise and for their passion regarding restoring people to good health.

Grace, Oakmont Pa

No Tylenol, No Tubes

Over the past ten years, I have been experiencing severe headaches, indulging in a bottle of Tylenol a month. Just a short five weeks later, NO medication, NO headaches and feeling great!

The kids had ear infection after ear infection. We were always at the pediatrician's for antibiotics. They had to have higher and higher doses and stronger antibiotics, giving them severe diarrhea and diaper rashes. After we were advised to have surgery for ear tubes AGAIN, a friend told us about chiropractic and how it worked for his family. I can happily say that since we've been under Dr. Tressler's care, we have been antibiotic-free! The ear infections are a thing of the past, and we've only had to go to the pediatrician for yearly check-ups! What a difference!

Kathleen Gary, Pittsburgh Pa

Overcoming Neck Surgeries

Before chiropractic adjustments, I had a very painful neck and limited mobility on my right side. I had two neck surgeries; which included five screws and two plates installed on my cervical spine. This was to alleviate pain. It didn't work.

I had to calculate every movement I made, even canceling my daily routines. Chiropractic care with Dr. Tressler on a weekly routine has vastly improved my quality of life beyond belief. I have lost weight, reduced the amount on medications I need, and have fewer visits to my MD.

Darnell Palmer, Pittsburgh Pa

My Hunt for Health

It still amazes me when God answers my prayers even when it happens so many times. The weight loss I have just experienced is nothing short of a true blessing. I spent thirty years as an administrator in the Pennsylvania Department of Corrections and was able to retire with a full pension and benefits at the age of fifty-two. What a wonderful blessing to be able to pursue any of my many passions. I am an avid outdoorsman, and I love to hunt and fish. I now work as a fly fishing guide, spending over 180 days a year fishing and experiencing the wonder and beauty that God created all around us. There was only one problem. After years of sitting behind a desk in a high stress occupation, my weight had ballooned to over 270 pounds.

I was still active but felt tired all the time. I never felt like I had any energy, and even though I did not want to admit it, my weight was affecting how I was enjoying life. I tried to diet and exercise but would gain and lose a few times a month, never making any progress. Exercise was very difficult at the weight I was, and because of that I hated to do it; so, I started to pray about my weight.

I mow the grass for my neighbor and one day realized that her appearance was different. I asked her if she had gotten a new hairdo. She said no but that she had lost 28 pounds on a new program she was on. My neighbor experiences many medical challenges; so, I know that she was not exercising, and I thought to myself, "If she could lose 28 pounds, I could lose 30 pounds." The thought of being 30 pounds lighter was very appealing. I asked her how she was doing it, and she told me about Dr. Tressler. I was busy guiding fishing trips and was not able to attend the weight loss seminar for about a month after I had received the information.
Finally, I called Dr. Tressler's office and made the appointment to go and hear about the program at a weight loss seminar.

Everything that was described that evening made a great deal of sense to me. I also felt that cleaning up my diet and the benefit of chiropractic adjustment might help both my wife and me. My wife had been experiencing debilitating headaches; so, the plan to help her with the headaches and help with my weight loss was a win-win proposition.

The plan designed for me called for me to pick a goal weight, and I was not sure what a realistic figure was. I put down 215 pounds, hoping to be able to lose even half of that. I was booked to go on an elk hunting trip in Colorado on October 5th. I started the program on September 12th and lost 20 pounds before my trip. It was easy, and I could see and feel the results. I was worried about gaining back the weight I lost while on my trip; so, I went on the maintenance phase of the program while I was traveling. I packed meals that covered every day I would be gone and used a calorie counting device on my phone. I was able to stick to my plan, and, to my surprise, I lost 5 pounds while on the maintenance phase. I went back on the turbo loss program after I returned from my trip, and my weight loss continued.

By the time deer season started in early December, I had lost 40 pounds and was feeling better than I had in years. My energy level had gone through the roof. I was climbing hills that in years past had nearly killed me. I enjoyed the hunt more than I have in a number of years. I was climbing trees, carrying my tree stand into areas I had not been able to hunt for years. The weight loss has changed my life and the quality of my life.

I take Coumadin for a blood disorder that made me have blood clots and in 2005 gave me bilateral pulmonary embolism that nearly took my life. Since that time, I had taken a large daily dose of medication. After three months on the plan, my medication has been cut in half.

So, the day of this writing is exactly three months since I started the program, December 12th. I am 56.7 pounds lighter, and I have reached my goal of 215 pounds. My quality of life is 100%

better. While on the program, I found out I am going to become a grandfather. In February, I will get a grandson. God is good! I want to be around to introduce my grandson to the woods and water. All of this is to the glory of God.

Barry Johnson, Indiana Pa

My Neighbor Changed My Life

Dr. Aaron Tressler defines commitment as his practical approach to health, fitness, and nutrition.

I have had the pleasure of knowing Dr. Tressler for over twenty years, first as his next-door neighbor and friend, then as a patient, and now as a follower of his active and fit lifestyle. Aaron's example of the consumption of whole food nutrition and a balance of exercise, along with a healthy dose of spiritual well-being, has changed my life.

I once weighed 275 pounds and was out of breath walking up a flight of stairs. Today, I weigh 210 pounds, exercise four to six days a week, run up stairs, and enjoy a confidence and health that are through the roof. As President and CEO of an international association, energy and drive are key components of what make me a success, and they were a benefit obtained when I started a healthily lifestyle as taught by Dr. Tressler.

Read this book over and over. It will help to change your life.

Greg Nemchick, Hempfield Pa
PRESIDENT/CEO
WorkPlace Furnishings

My Little Girl

Since Autumn was six months old, we've been taking her to the eye doctor. They told us that by the time she was eight or nine she would be nearsighted. They could tell just by the exam of her eyes.

We started bringing Autumn to Dr. Tressler when she was four years old, and she has had perfect vision ever since. She is thirteen now and still is the only one of my five children who has perfect vision. The eye doctor is amazed and has told us to keep doing what we've been doing because it works. I have Autumn's eye exam to prove all of this.

Thanks, Dr. T.

God Bless,
Kelly, Jeannette Pa

Livin' on a Prayer

I would like to share my story of the inspiration I received as your program has helped to turn around my physical well-being.

In September of 2013, my weight and physical condition had deteriorated to the point where I was approaching 300 pounds for the first time in my life. My wife, Mary Jo, encouraged me to call and attend your meeting, and I did and decided to take it upon myself to make a change in what I was doing.

Since October, I have lost over 40 pounds (officially 36 pounds according to Sandy), and I am beginning Phase 2 next week to take this thing to another level and towards long-term health and well-being. For that, I thank you and your staff, for your commitment to the program and helping me achieve part of my goal.

As Jon Bon Jovi sings in his popular hit, "I am halfway there and livin' on a prayer." If you ask many people I know, they'd tell you that they wouldn't have given me a prayer to do the program. I thank you for proving them wrong and providing an easy way of understanding what needs to be done and giving me a second chance. I have thirty to forty more pounds to go, and I have no doubt that it will happen.

Awesome!

Jeff Mauro, Murrysville Pa

Help! My Boy Can't Breathe

Chiropractic has saved my son, Sebastian, with asthma and allergies. He is 6 ½ years old. At 5 ½ months, he was diagnosed with respiratory syncytial virus (RSV).

I watched my son be put into an oxygen tent and given multiple doses of steroids and Albuterol, asthma medications that help to reduce swelling in the chest walls and keep the airways open to allow for proper air flow to stop wheezing and gasping for air. We spent three days under these conditions and were sent home with a nebulizer in hand and all of the medications to go with it.

I can't count the number of treatments my son went through. He has had the croup six times since the age of one. He has been rushed to the hospital with severe asthma attacks more than nine times, even with the use of Albuterol through the nebulizer and a fast-acting inhaler. He has been on steroids more than five times, sometimes for ten-day periods and once for an entire summer.

Sebastian suffered a very traumatic birth. He was delivered naturally but needed a vacuum assist. He had stopped breathing after my first push, and the doctor could not wait for his head any longer. He was literally sucked out during my second push in order to save his life. Not until my son was four years old did I hear a seminar on chiropractic and its benefits. I had taken him off of the preventative medications three months prior to seeking alternative means and tried specialty type shakes and diet changes to help his body rid itself of the yeast that had built up after so many years of antibiotics, but I did not feel that was enough since we were still seeking emergency medical help due to sudden asthma attacks and other respiratory illnesses.

Finally, I decided to give chiropractic a try. When Sebastian was first x-rayed, I was astonished at what I saw. His neck had actually been reversed, and he had two severe subluxations of his upper neck and back. The bones were touching one another. Dr. Tressler was convinced that this was the result of his traumatic birth. You see, this is not how the back or neck is supposed to be. Each bone is to be evenly spaced apart. I looked at a diagram from high school Biology, showing me the central nervous system and what organ or organs each nerve attends to. Believe it or not, the vertebrae in Sebastian's neck that were subluxated actually housed the nerves that run to the lungs!

Ever since that amazing revelation, Sebastian has been under the chiropractic care of Dr. Aaron Tressler. Periodic x-rays were and are being taken to show his progress. His neck is finally moving into the correct position, and the two vertebrae that were touching have actually separated. We have not made a hospital visit in more than a year, and he has been off all medications. Sebastian has not gotten any type of respiratory, bacterial or viral infection in more than a year. I attribute this to his chiropractic care and diet. This all proves to me that chiropractic care has a healthier, more positive effect on the body than antibiotics for chronic illnesses.

Remember, your body is a machine. You have the ability to keep it healthy. You make the choice!

Toni Maione, Irwin Pa

Cross-Eyed at Birth

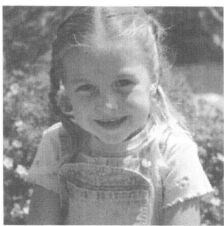

Sydney Tressler, Dr. Tressler's 4th daughter

Having five children, I have had many experiences with health-related issues that I had to deal with, understand, and overcome. One of the most interesting of all my stories started when my fourth daughter, Sydney, was born. Sydney, now twelve years old, was born at home with our midwife, with no complications; however, within hours after birth, we noticed that her right eye was drawing towards the middle, appearing cross-eyed. I had already checked her for subluxation minutes after birth and all appeared well; so, I began investigating other areas to explain why her eye was still crossed. I found her right cranial bones had shifted out of position (due to the birth process) and were fixated.

Newborns' cranial bones are movable to allow the cranium to go through the birth canal more easily. There are soft spots, the sutures, which allow this to happen. I gently began to adjust (slide) the cranial bone by very gently stroking this locked bone to the right position, and BAM, her eye sprung back like it was attached to a rubber band. I continued this for eight straight days, and each day it kept improving. After eight days, it was fixed. I have never seen anything this traumatic in a child in all my years of practice. Birth trauma can occur in many ways, and all children need to be examined before permanent subluxation and damage occurs.

Sydney actually had strabismus, not a lazy eye. Strabismus is when an eye is weak and crosses to the middle. When an eye is crossed, the child gets a different picture from each eye. The child's brain blocks out the picture from the weaker eye. If the eye is not fixed when a child is young (under six is the critical stage), the child's brain will always ignore the pictures from the weak eye! The first few years of life are critical for proper neurological development, which develops a child mentally, physically, and behaviorally. So, a crossed-eye could lead to developmental weakness and less than 100% development of language and hand/eye coordination, mental confusion, and just less than their God-given potential.

Having learned this information, I knew it was crucial for Sydney to have "normal" eyes. What was in her future? An eye patch, hours of therapy, special glasses, or even surgery? All of these may have to be considered, but thank God, her eye returned to normal. Sydney continues to get straight A's and is incredibly smart and a fantastic athlete. This would have been destroyed if her vision was altered.

My office works with one of the top specialists in the area, Dr. Hans Lessman, who, with the latest technology, helps restore these eye problems naturally, without surgery. His work is magnificent, and his results are even better. If you have a child with a weak or cross-eye, or even know someone with this problem, have a proper chiropractic exam immediately, and visit Dr. Lessman to have this problem resolved now before it becomes too late.

Dr. Aaron Tressler – dad.

Complete Family Health

Our family has been patients of Dr. Tressler's practice for several years. I can tell you that we have seen a distinct difference in our health. Our kids, who are now 17, 15 and 13, were young children when we first starting see him.

They would get ear infections, Strep throat, the flu – nothing outrageous but we would all get sick a few times a year. I was just thinking the other day that we have not been sick once in the past couple of years – not once. Then I thought about the time and money it has save us in doctor's visits, trips to the pharmacy and missing work and school. But more importantly, it feels amazing to be healthy. We are very grateful to have found a chiropractor who takes such good care of us and keeps us feeling great!

Jeff & Beth Scanio & Family, Harrison City Pa

Antibiotics, Allergies and Apparatus ... Oh My!

"Why don't we just put tubes in his ears?" was the question that finally drove us to try chiropractic care. At eighteen months old, Caleb already had enough to deal with. He was allergic to wheat, barley, eggs, milk, corn, soy, nuts, cats, dogs, dust mites, and several other things. In addition, he was on several medications for asthma and allergies and frequently needed breathing treatments. Our older son, Zachary, shared these later issues with Caleb.

Caleb began having ear infections very frequently, so frequently that when we would go to the pediatrician for his three-week ear check-up, he would have another ear infection. That meant course after course after course of antibiotics. At that point, we thought we might as well "try" chiropractic care.

Within weeks of beginning chiropractic care, we took Caleb off all medications, and he no longer required breathing treatments. His sensitivity to many allergens has greatly decreased. And the ear infections? He never had another one again! He will be four next month, and this simple decision has already greatly increased the quality of his life.

In addition, Zachary is also off of all medications, and he has never needed another breathing treatment. Come to think of it, I forget where that machine is located now!

My husband, Josh, had chronic sinus infections, which required several courses of antibiotics every winter, and now he no longer has these infections at all! We both sleep better and have very few headaches. We discovered, when we had our x-rays, that my spine looked like a "C" when looking at me from the front. Now my spine is virtually perfect.

There is one negative to chiropractic care. We get sick so infrequently that it becomes VERY irritating the few times we do get sick. But then, we just come see Dr. Tressler a few extra times that week!!

When I saw my son's pediatrician last month for his regular check-up, he commented to me, "You know, over the past two years, I have only seen you for the yearly check-ups. I was used to seeing you so frequently."

I just smiled and thought to myself, "Two years, that is exactly how long we have been going to Dr. Tressler for chiropractic care."

The Lorenz Family, Murrysville Pa

Mom's Broken Heart Stayed the Course

Here is our story: As a new mother, I approached my children's health the same way that my parents had approached my health. For prevention of disease, we vaccinated according to the schedule recommended by the Center for Disease Control (CDC) and went to the pediatrician for advice and ultimately to resolve the problem. When my daughter was sick, which was a lot more frequently than I was sick as an infant and child, we gave her Tylenol for fevers and would receive vaccines, as the doctor recommended.

When she was sick, often with earaches, we gave her antibiotics, even though we were uncertain if the cause were bacterial or viral. During the fall, my daughter turned one year old and had three earaches between October and December and was on three types of antibiotics for them. In February, she had another ear infection, and we took her to the emergency room because she was having trouble breathing. That was the first time my daughter was diagnosed with asthma. I was in shock. How could this be? Neither my husband nor I had asthma, and there was no history of it in our families. We were clueless about the underlying cause of asthma and did what the medical doctors said to treat asthma with an inhaler and steroids.

Meanwhile, I was pregnant with our second child who, within the first six weeks of birth, was having trouble breastfeeding and was very irritable and spitting up. The pediatrician thought it might be acid reflux; so, we started her on some antacid medicine, and when she improved, the diagnosis was confirmed.

She seemed to be developing fine, yet, at her 15 month vaccinations and her 18 month vaccinations she had bad reactions. The first time, she had an extremely high fever, was moaning, turned pale white, and lost her coordination.

Because her high fever did not occur on the days listed on the VIS page, the doctors did not consider the fever associated with a vaccine reaction. Over the next several weeks, she gradually and gratefully regained her coordination. I do not know why I vaccinated again at 18 months, but all I can say is that I completely trusted the medical system and could not understand how it might not work for a child's best interest. Again, at her 18 month vaccinations, my daughter had a bad reaction with high fever which was again disregarded by her doctors. In addition to losing her coordination again, she was severely constipated where she had to strain in pain for half an hour and a red face to pass a bowel movement.

It was quite frightening to watch this. Never before from a medical practitioner had I heard of constipation as a reaction to vaccines, but it can be because the toxins are trying to be purged through the intestines.

Jump forward six months after a summer of moving twice and vacations, and my oldest daughter is about to turn four and my second daughter is two years old. Both daughters are facing a myriad of behavioral problems including hyperactivity, insomnia, gagging reaction to foods, bad bellyaches, itchiness, tantrums, sweating, and bad dreams. As a mom, I was in a very dark place. I was lost and desperate, extremely stressed, not understanding why my children were sick and unhappy.

Our medical doctor ran tests that didn't show any allergies. She thought that the behavioral issues were related to the stress of moving and suggested we see a psychiatrist. I knew in my gut that these symptoms were a physiological problem, not a psychological one. I remember lying on my bed in the dark, weeping while my oldest daughter laid screaming and thrashing in bed next door, unable to sleep and in pain. At that moment, I pleaded and asked God to please help me out of this mess, to show me the way, knowing that He is the only one who can do this.

I began to read a book I had randomly purchased on Amazon six months earlier, *Healing the New Childhood Epidemics: Autism, ADHD, Allergies, and Asthma*. This was the first time that I read anything about asthma and how it is an autoimmune disease......what I read clicked and made sense. These readings lead me to the only DAN (Defeat Autism Now) doctor in our area who was a chiropractor. I had never been to a chiropractor before, and we got in for an appointment as soon as possible. I was a sponge soaking up all I could.

We began making changes to our diet, including eliminating major allergens, eating organic vegetables and grass-fed meats, and we started getting adjusted and taking supplements. We reduced toxins in our home and food. Within six months of these initial changes, my oldest daughter was offer asthma medication, and my second daughter was off her medicine for acid reflux. In addition, tantrums were almost non-existent, and hyperactivity was gone. God was answering my prayer.

Looking back, I realize that I had been putting my faith in the medical doctors above my faith in God. God gives us medical doctors on earth to help us, but putting doctors on a pedestal next to God is not healthy. I trusted man more than I trusted God. I trusted doctors who did not know my children or me more than I trusted myself with God's help to take care of my children.

I trusted medicine to solve the health problems of my family more than I trusted the innate God-given potential of our miraculous bodies and immune system to heal and fight disease. I was not treating my body or the bodies of my children as temples of God.....I had been polluting our bodies with toxins contributing to our poor health and behavioral problems. I was

119

just like the majority of Americans who get vaccinated, eat processed foods and a high sugar diet, don't worry about pesticides or toxins in the home, and use antibiotics and medicine routinely to treat symptoms. Traditional western medicine and the American lifestyle led us on a downward spiral. Making a paradigm shift to a chiropractic model of health and nutrition may be countercultural, but it is the best thing I did to promote the long-term health of our family.

Be strong, be open-minded to a new healthy paradigm, make small continuous changes to your lifestyle, and you will see positive long-term results!

Dr. Tressler and his staff have been the blessing to our long journey. We understand now that this course we are on will be successful. It will have some rough roads, but nothing like we would have through a life of drugs, hospitals and psychiatrists. The support we have at Tressler Chiropractic is just what will get us through. Thanks.

Sara and Adam Schaut, Murrysville Pa

From Cancer to Conqueror

It all started after college, and went downhill from there. A collegiate athlete, having to go through 4 knee surgeries, later on became a mother of two. Pregnancies were not easy and had me off my feet for the majority of the time. So my lack of mobility du e to my knees and pregnancy made it real easy for the weight to just pile on and on and on.

If that wasn't enough, I was diagnosed with cervical cancer late in my second pregnancy. After my youngest son was born I had to have a radical hysterectomy. Although that wasn't the end, the cancer had come back 2 years later requiring me to enter an intense chemo and radiation therapy treatment.

After the years of fighting, I was told I was back in good health and yet, I felt anything but healthy. I couldn't sit on the floor because of knee pain, migraines were a common ailment, working out of my home I suffered with lower back and neck pain and I didn't know what it meant to have a good night sleep. I was no longer myself, my disposition was that of a miserable person. I was always on edge, snapping at my family at the smallest things, and by 8:00 at night I was ready for bed. So, I may have been home for my kids but was I really getting to enjoy my family the way God intended?

One day, as I was praying for a change in me, I was listening to the radio and cried with hopelessness then God answered my prayer. I heard Dr. Tressler and his words spoke to me enough to make an appointment. Here I am 5 months later and I am back to the person I longed to be once again!

Not only have I lost 60 pounds (37 lbs. in the first 40 days of the program) I am enjoying my family once again, I can run a little more with my boys, we can camp out on the floor and watch movies. Overall I am much happier and much more patient. I havent experienced in a migraine in months and my energy level has skyrocketed! And because of this I am a much more productive person and member of my family.

Because of the positive affect Dr. Tressler, his staff and his program has had on me I am LIVING LIFE! I am not just getting through it day by day. Now my boys are receiving chiropractic care from Dr. T and the changes in them have been just as positive! We are a family that is LIVING our lives to the FULLEST!

Thank you Dr. T and all the amazing staff that have helped me succeed in my journey to a better me!

Christine Gallagher, Greensburg Pa

Cancer? My scans are clear!

I am Donna Z., and I thank God every day for leading me to Dr. T. and showing me the way to overcome my health problems.

In December 2012, after surgery for a total hysterectomy, I was diagnosed with high-grade endometrial cancer. Of the people who get endometrial cancer only about 10% get this type. It was described as aggressive and able to travel outside the uterus. The recommended treatment was six rounds of chemo followed by radiation. Since there is little data regarding this type of cancer, the estimated outcome after treatment was a 50% chance that treatment would eliminate the cancer or that the cancer would not recur. This did not sound promising, along with the fact that it would kill healthy cells, compromise my immune system even more, and went against all I believe.

I believe God created a perfect body with the ability to heal itself and that He gave me everything I need to make this happen. I also know, based on over sixty years of lifestyle, that diet and environment have taken a toll. Now, with a cancer diagnosis, I needed to take action to restore my body and give it a chance to do what God intended it to do -- heal. Dr. T. was eager to help me conquer the cancer and regain optimal health.

With regular adjustments, home spinal rehab therapy, vitamin D3, and a predominately plant based diet that includes approximately forty ounces of fresh vegetable juice a day, and a positive attitude – I started healing. In February 2013, seven weeks after my diagnosis, I had a CT scan. Seven hours after the scan, my oncologist called to say the scans were clear. Clear scans and twenty-two pounds lighter – time for a "happy dance."

It is now December 2013 twelve months after my journey with cancer began. In this time, I have found that not only have I gotten healthier but I have also attained victory in areas I have struggled in for many years. I have also come to believe this lifestyle is effective no matter what health challenge you face. It is also a wonderful way to avoid health issues in the future. I have won my battle with weight, dropping twenty-five pounds to date and keeping it off with not one thought of diet.

At the age of sixty-one, I find my skin has great color and glows. I searched for years for the right diet, cream, powder or potion to attain these goals (with little to no success) only to find them to be the side effect of cleaning up my act. I have more energy for spending time with my family, especially my grandchildren, and to me there is no greater joy.

I thank God for creating the perfect body (a body that will heal itself) and everything needed for it to do just that. I also give thanks for His grace in showing me the way to do this. My God is amazing and faithful to all His promises; so, even though I am a work in process, I know He gives me the strength and determination to overcome every challenge.

Donna Z, Plum Boro Pa

Real life, real people – those are their testimonies – men, women, moms, dads, grandfathers, and grandmothers, laborers, professionals, people of various ages, the guy next door.

Throughout this book, I've given you the facts about the ABC's of health, and now I have let you hear the hearts of the folks who have put them into practice in their daily lives.

So, where do you go from here? You need to realize that all kinds of people from all walks of life and demographics, even children and infants, are living below their God-ordained potential, are sick, and are even dying. Why is this so? Our Maker knows why. He says, *My people perish (are destroyed) for a lack of knowledge (Hosea 4:6).*

That verse has many applications, one of them being health, even the health of God's own children. Contrary to the popular saying, ignorance is NOT bliss. Ignorance can rob you of your health and even kill you even though your Father has a better plan in mind.

I know these are sobering thoughts, but the good news is that YOU are no longer ignorant. You have this book in your hand, and that means you have knowledge. You now know your ABC's, can refer back to them again and again, and you can put them into practice, just like Alice, Anita, Donna, Barry, Shirley, John, Sandy, and so many others have done. Trust in God first, follow their example, and put your knowledge of the ABC's into practice. Then, you can appropriate God's heartfelt desire for you:

With long life will I satisfy you and show you My salvation (Psalm 91:16).

See, I set before you today life and prosperity, death and destruction. For I command you today to love the Lord your God, to walk in his ways, and to keep his commands, decrees, and laws; then you will live and increase, and the Lord your God will bless you in the land you are entering to posses.
Deuteronomy 30:15-16

It can't end with a more appropriate verse. Take that verse to heart and apply it. Your life will change.

God bless, Dr. T

26018020R00071

Made in the USA
Charleston, SC
22 January 2014